The Renal System Explained

An illustrated core text

Sunita R. Deshmukh, BMedSci (Hons)
Fourth Year Medical Student
Faculty of Medicine and Health Sciences, University of Nottingham, UK

Newton W.K. Wong, BMedSci (Hons)
Fourth Year Medical Student
Faculty of Medicine and Health Sciences, University of Nottingham, UK

Nottingham University Press

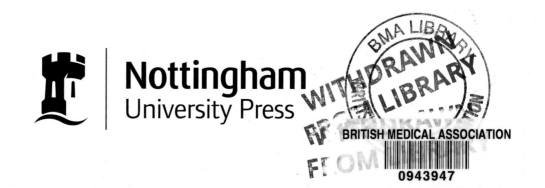

Nottingham University Press
Manor Farm, Main Street, Thrumpton
Nottingham, NG11 0AX, United Kingdom
www.nup.com

NOTTINGHAM

First published 2009
© SR Deshmukh and NWK Wong

British Library Cataloguing in Publication Data
The Renal System Explained - An illustrated core text
I. Deshmukh, S.R; II. Wong, N.W.K.

ISBN 978-1-904761-84-6

Disclaimer

Every reasonable effort has been made to ensure that the material in this book is true, correct, complete and appropriate at the time of writing. Nevertheless the publishers, the editors and the authors do not accept responsibility for any omission or error, or for any injury, damage, loss or financial consequences arising from the use of the book.

FIGURE CREDITS

Original diagrams and front cover
Sunita R. Deshmukh

Original photography
Dr. Susan Anderson
Newton W. K. Wong

Figures 3.3, 3.18 and 5.13 reprinted with permission from Alan Stevens, James Lowe and Ian Scott.
Core pathology, 3rd ed. Mosby, Copyright Elsevier (2008).

Typeset by Nottingham University Press, Nottingham
Printed and bound by H. Charlesworth & Co Ltd, Wakefield

CONTENTS

DEDICATIONS

For their unconditional love and support, I dedicate this book to my family, who have been my inspiration and to whom I owe everything:

To my parents, Rohini & Rajiv
and my brother, Sandeep

In loving memory of my brother, Deepak
and my grandparents, Asha & Ganesh and Raj Rani & Murari Lal.

Thanks also to my colleague Newton Wong, for initiating this project.

Sunita R. Deshmukh

The figures in this book could not have been possible without the tremendous talent of my dear friend and co-author Sunita Deshmukh, and I would like to say a big thank you for her dedication and hard work on the manuscript as a whole. My pursuit of medicine is made possible by my parents and brother, and I thank them for their love and all that they have done. In addition, I would also like to express my gratitude to Dr. C. K. Liu, MD a family physician in Toronto, Canada whose wise words of wisdom and character inspires me and is the epitome of a true physician.

Newton W. K. Wong

Contributors

Faculty Advisors

Professor James S. Lowe, BMedSci, BMBS, DM, FRCPath
Associate Dean of Medical Education,
Professor of Neuropathology and Honorary Consultant Histopathologist
Faculty of Medicine and Health Sciences, University of Nottingham, UK

Professor Terry M. Mayhew, BA (Oxon), PhD
Professor of Anatomy,
Faculty of Medicine and Health Sciences, University of Nottingham, UK

Dr. Vera Ralevic, BSc, PhD
Associate Professor and Reader in Cardiovascular Sciences,
Renal & Endocrine Systems Module Convenor,
Faculty of Medicine and Health Sciences, University of Nottingham, UK

Dr. Michael D. Randall, MA, PhD
Associate Professor and Reader in Cardiovascular Pharmacology,
Faculty of Medicine and Health Sciences, University of Nottingham, UK

Student Contributors

Sandeep R. Deshmukh, BA (Hons)
Final Year Medical Student,
Trinity College, University of Cambridge, UK

Ch. 3: Structure of the Renal System

Iram Haneef, BMedSci (Hons)
Fourth Year Medical Student,
Faculty of Medicine and Health Sciences, University of Nottingham, UK

Ch. 3: Structure of the Renal System

Acknowledgements

The authors are grateful to the following individuals in the Faculty of Medicine & Health Sciences at the University of Nottingham, for their help in the preparation of the anatomical and histological photographs used in this textbook: **Dr. Susan Anderson** (Advanced Microscopy Unit) and **Ryan J. Thachen-Cary, MSc** (Prosector and Dissection Room Manager). Thanks also to **Dr. Rakesh H. Ganatra** (Consultant Radiologist and Nuclear Medicine Physician) for his advice on Appendix 2 – Clinical Imaging Overview.

PREFACE

Co-authoring a textbook has been an exciting and challenging learning curve in our young careers – especially alongside our ongoing clinical course!

The renal system is an incredible instrument of mammalian homeostasis, exploiting a remarkable array of bio-physico-chemical mechanisms to maintain a multitude of functions. That said, not all students will necessarily have the time, desire or need to fully appreciate all the intricate fascinations this system has to offer. So we embarked upon this project to create a learning resource comprised of clear and concise explanations of key concepts. This book contains core knowledge, identifies and emphasises essential learning points, and also enables readers to explore additional information if they are so inclined. It is primarily written for pre-clinical undergraduate students but also serves as a comprehensive guide for clinical students and a reference for science professionals.

'The Renal System Explained' offers the exam-going student's perspective as well as the expertise of experienced, specialist contributors. Appraisals of the manuscript, from students and academic professionals, have been a source of great encouragement and guidance throughout the process. We hope the final publication inspires student interest in the renal system and supports exam preparation.

Sunita R. Deshmukh & Newton W. K. Wong

KEY FEATURES

Detailed contents at beginning of book

Summarised contents at beginning of each chapter

Integrative case study at end of each chapter

Exam-style self-assessment questions at end of each chapter

Clear, concise and colourful figures and tables throughout

Appendices with overviews of clinical aspects

Information boxes

Colour-coded boxes are used to categorise and present information in an easily accessible, clear and concise way. Headings identify the type of information contained within each box:

KEY POINTS

These boxes highlight important facts and concepts related to a specific topic. The primary text is a background for the *Key points*, which serve as chapter learning objectives designed to aid exam preparation.

ASK YOURSELF

These short-answer questions promote critical thinking, application of acquired knowledge and understanding, as well as facilitating exam preparation.

REMEMBER !

These boxes present basic facts or concepts to learn and always bear in mind. They appear at relevant points in the text, unlike *Key points* boxes which summarise information at the end of a section.

POINTS OF INTEREST

These boxes compliment core reading and aid understanding of broad terms. Although *Points of interest* are not crucial for exam preparation, introducing ideas beyond the limits of core text may help students remember key information.

CLINICAL RELEVANCE

Clinical relevance covers relevant aspects of pathology and pharmacology, with emphasis on morphological and/or physiological significance. This includes information regarding the pathological basis of disease processes (aetiology and pathogenesis). In-depth discussion of clinical management is generally avoided.

CHAPTER 1 — BODY FLUID BALANCE

Written by: Sunita Deshmukh

The concepts covered in this chapter are all fundamental aspects of the renal system. This system is designed, structurally (anatomically) and functionally (physiologically), to handle fluids within the body in a highly efficient way. Water is the most abundant component of the human body, accounting for roughly two-thirds of the average person's body weight. The physicochemical processes responsible for maintaining fluid and electrolyte homeostasis in the human body are vital. An awareness of the underlying regulatory mechanisms is also important when considering various pathological changes.

The basic principles are relatively simple to remember and apply, provided you have a clear understanding of them from the outset. The core material in this chapter forms a good starting point for studying the renal system as its relevance can be appreciated throughout.

BODY FLUID DISTRIBUTION

Body fluid compartments

Intracellular and extracellular fluid

Fluid is compartmentalised in the body as shown in Figure 1.1. Body fluid volume and distribution can vary with age, gender and proportion of body fat, since adipose tissue has a low water content compared with other tissues (see *Points of interest 1.1*).

The two major divisions of body fluid are separated by the cell membrane:

- **Intracellular fluid (ICF)** – contains a relatively large volume within the body's cells (about two-thirds of total body water)

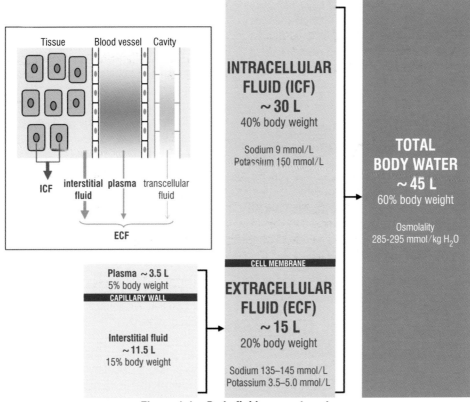

Figure 1.1 – Body fluid compartments

- **Extracellular fluid (ECF)** – smaller volume of fluid outside cells (about one-third of total body water).

The ECF is further sub-divided into two major compartments, separated by the capillary endothelium, and a minor compartment:

- **Interstitial fluid** – occupies the space between cells and outside capillaries (makes up about two-thirds of ECF volume)

- **Plasma** – the non-cellular part of blood, found inside capillaries i.e. intravascular (plasma accounts for about a third of ECF volume)

- **Transcellular fluid** – contains only a small amount of water, including epithelial secretions such as synovial, pericardial, intraocular and cerebrospinal fluid.

Transcellular fluid is said to occupy a 'third space' (3 extracellular fluid compartments in total). Minor compartments of body fluid, like lymph and transcellular (third space) fluids are negligible in terms of their quantitative contribution to ECF.

The major fluid compartments of the body, with average values for volume and percentage of total body weight. are shown in Figure 1.1.

CLINICAL RELEVANCE 1.1

In pharmacology, the **volume of distribution (V_d)** of a drug is defined as the apparent volume of fluid in which the total dose of the drug is distributed at the same concentration as in the plasma. This value is useful in dosage calculations such as loading doses. Generally the following can be assumed about the nature of drug distribution, based on our knowledge of body fluid compartments (Fig.1.1):

V_d = 3 L	drug only in plasma
V_d = 14 L	drug in plasma and interstitial fluid i.e. ECF
V_d = 40–45 L	drug occupying total body water i.e. ICF + ECF
V_d > 45 L	drug widely distributed and extensively bound in body tissues

Blood volume

Blood has intracellular (blood cells) and extracellular (plasma) fluid components, contained intravascularly within the circulation. The fraction of total blood volume that is composed of red blood cells is known as the 'packed cell volume' (PCV) or haematocrit. The significance of this value in assessing renal disease is explained in *Clinical relevance 1.2*.

The total blood volume can be calculated from known values of haematocrit and plasma volume, as shown in equation 1.1, using typical values for a normal adult. Plasma volume is measured using serum albumin labelled with radioactive iodine, or less commonly by injecting a dye that binds to plasma proteins in the circulation.

$$\text{Total blood volume} = \frac{\text{Plasma volume}}{1 - \text{Haematocrit}}$$

$$5\,\text{L} = \frac{3\,\text{L}}{1 - 0.4} \tag{1.1}$$

CLINICAL RELEVANCE 1.2

PCV, or haematrocrit, can be calculated from known values of:

- Red blood cell count

- Mean corpuscular volume (MCV) i.e. the average volume of a red blood cell.

Calculation of PCV is shown in equation 1.2 using approximate average values for a normal adult. Normal ranges are provided in Appendix 3 (haematocrit 0.42–0.45).

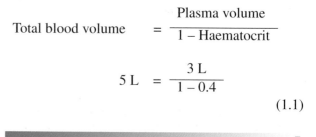

$$\text{Mean corpuscular volume} \times \text{Red blood cell count} = \text{Haematocrit}$$

$$90 \times 10^{-15}\,\text{L} \times 5 \times 10^{12}/\text{L} = 0.45\ (45\%\ \text{of total blood volume}) \tag{1.2}$$

Polycythaemia is characterised by an abnormally raised concentration of red blood cells (erythrocytes), usually accompanied by increased levels of haemoglobin and PCV. Haemoglobin levels may be affected by other conditions (physiological and pathological e.g. iron-deficiency), therefore clinically PCV is a more reliable indicator of polycythaemia.

Changes in PCV may reflect:

- A change in the actual volume of red blood cells
- A change in the total blood volume.

In **absolute polycythaemia** the red blood cell volume is raised, whereas **relative polycythaemia** occurs due to a fall in plasma volume (the actual volume of red cells remains normal, but the concentration rises).

Absolute polycythaemia may have a primary or secondary underlying cause. Primary polycythaemia (**polycythaemia rubra vera**, or erythrocytosis) is an example of a myeloproliferative disorder (uncontrolled clonal proliferation of bone marrow cell lines). Absolute polycythaemia may be secondary to high levels of erythropoietin, the primary stimulus for erythrocyte production. Causes may be:

- Physiological e.g. high-altitude living
- Pathological e.g. diseases of the kidney that inappropriately increase the secretion of erythropoietin, lung disease, cyanotic heart disease.

Water as a percentage of body weight, is influenced by age, gender and percentage of body fat. Body water percentage is highest in neonates and decreases to the normal average adult value of $\sim$60% by one year of age. Body water percentage is typically lower in women than in men because women have a higher percentage of body fat (due to actions of the female sex hormone oestrogen).

REMEMBER !

Water content in adipose tissue is low, relative to water content in other tissue types.

Constituents of body fluid

The ionic compositions of the ICF and ECF differ considerably, due to the low electrolyte permeability of the highly selective cell membrane that divides these two fluid compartments. The electrolyte composition of each body fluid compartment is predominated by a particular ion:

- ECF – Sodium ions (Na^+)
- ICF – Potassium ions (K^+).

Both of these cations are accompanied by their attendant anions:

- ECF – the major anions accompanying Na^+ are **Cl^- and HCO_3^-**
- ICF – K^+ is accompanied primarily by **PO_4^{3-}** (as well as negatively charged cellular proteins which cannot escape the cell).

ECF compartments (plasma and interstitial fluid) are only separated by capillary endothelium which is freely permeable to small ions, so their ionic compositions are similar. The important difference between the two major ECF compartments is the relatively high plasma concentration of plasma proteins, which tend to remain in the capillary due to its low permeability to these proteins.

REMEMBER !

Na^+ is the predominant cation of the ECF and K^+ is the major cation of the ICF (Fig. 1.1).

ASK YOURSELF 1.1 ?

Q. What is the physiological significance of the difference in Na^+ and K^+ distribution between the extracellular and intracellular fluid?

A. The uneven distribution of Na^+, K^+ and large protein anions (as well as the differential membrane permeability to these ions) are responsible for:

Table 1.1 – ECF and external environment: processes of transfer between internal and external environment

Site of transfer	Input (to ECF)	Output (from ECF)
Digestive tract	Ingestion	Defecation
Lungs	Inspiration	Expiration
Body surface	Absorption through skin or mucosal surface, by injection	Perspiration, lacrimation, open wound (haemorrhage)

Table 1.2 – ECF and other internal sites: processes of transfer

Internal processes	Input (to ECF)	Output (from ECF)
Metabolism	Production	Consumption (irreversible)
Storage depots	Retrieval of stored constituents for temporary restoration of their plasma concentration	Storage of excess constituents for temporary maintenance of their normal plasma concentration
Reversible incorporation into more complex structures	Retrieval of ECF constituent	Removal of constituent from ECF by its conversion

1

- Resting cell membrane potential (separation of opposite charges across the plasma membrane)
- Generation of action potentials in excitable tissues (nerve and muscle cells) via changes in these variables.

ECF 'reservoir'

The concentrations of different substances in the ECF vary. The ECF acts as a readily available internal reservoir of its constituent substances. Transfer of substances can occur between the ECF and the external environment or between the ECF and other internal sites, via a number of exchange mechanisms summarised in Table 1.1 and Table 1.2.

Storage depots of ECF constituents have a limited capacity, therefore processes of transfer between the ECF (the body's internal reservoir) and other internal sites can only temporarily compensate for deviations in the normal plasma levels of ECF constituents.

> **REMEMBER** !
>
> Ultimately the maintenance of a stable balance of ECF constituents relies on the following equation:
>
> **TOTAL BODY INPUT = TOTAL BODY OUTPUT**
>
> This in turn depends on:
>
> - Exchanges between the ECF and the external environment i.e. the balance between ingestion and excretion
> - Metabolism i.e. the balance between anabolism (synthesis) and catabolism (breakdown) of ECF constituents.

> **KEY POINTS 1.1** 🗝
>
> Table 1.3 provides a summary of the normal volume and distribution of body fluids, given a total body water volume of 45 L.
>
> Total body water in a normal healthy adult is 40–45 L on average, accounting for 60% of body weight.
>
> The ICF and ECF are divided by the highly selective plasma membrane.
>
> Major differences between the ICF and ECF include:

- Presence of cellular proteins in the ICF, that cannot leave cells
- Unequal distribution of Na^+ and K^+ (and their accompanying anions).

Table 1.3 – Summary of the major body fluid compartments

Body fluid compartment	Volume (and as a fraction of total body fluid volume)
Intracellular fluid (ICF)	30 L ($^2/_3$)
Extracellular fluid (ECF)	15 L ($^1/_3$)

ECF component	Distribution	Volume (and as a fraction of total ECF volume)
Interstitial fluid	Outside the capillary, bathing cells	11.5 L ($\sim^3/_4$)
Plasma	Inside the capillary i.e. contained within blood vessels	3.5 L ($\sim^1/_4$)

> **REMEMBER** !
>
> The ICF is characterised by a relatively high concentration of potassium ions (K^+) i.e. 150 mmol/L.
>
> The ECF is characterised by:
>
> - Relatively high sodium ion (Na^+) concentration i.e. 135–145 mmol/L
> - Low K^+ concentration i.e. 3.5–5.0 mmol/L.
>
> The ECF compartments are separated by the highly permeable capillary endothelium.
>
> The main difference between ECF compartments is the higher concentration of plasma proteins in the blood plasma (only a small amount of plasma proteins leak into the interstitial fluid).
>
> The regulation of ECF constituents is summarised by the balance concept, which applies to the long-term balance of any substance within the body:
>
> **TOTAL BODY INPUT = TOTAL BODY OUTPUT**
>
> When input > output a POSITIVE balance exists
> When output > input a NEGATIVE balance exists

GENERAL PRINCIPLES OF FLUID BALANCE

The basic principles are explained before considering their physiological significance in regulating body fluid balance.

Electrolyte solutions

Concentration

> **REMEMBER** !
>
> The concentration of a substance in solution is defined as the amount of solute dissolved in a certain volume of solvent:
>
> $$\text{Concentration} = \frac{\text{Amount}}{\text{Volume}} \qquad (1.3)$$

Molarity (or molar concentration) is the amount of a substance relative to its molecular weight, and this can either be determined by dividing the mass of a substance by its molecular weight, or by dividing the number of moles by the volume of solution (see equation 1.4). Molarity is typically used to express the concentration of uncharged molecules (see *Points of interest 1.2*).

$$\text{Molarity} = \frac{\text{Number of moles}}{\text{Volume}} \qquad (1.4)$$

A **mole** (mol) of any substance is based on Avogadro's number (approximately 6.02×10^{23}) of the constituent entities of that substance. In contrast, the **osmole** (Osm) is a unit of measure for the total number of particles in a solution. Thus osmoles refer to the number of osmotically active (dissociable) particles in solution.

Osmolal concentration: osmolarity versus osmolality

Osmolal concentration is determined by the number of osmoles in a given volume or mass. Osmolal concentration is expressed in terms of either osmolarity or osmolality.

The key difference between osmolarity and osmolality lies in the different units of measure:

- Osmolarity – concentration expressed as osmoles per litre of solvent (Osm/L)
- Osmolality – concentration in osmoles per kilogram of solvent (Osm/kg).

The volume of a solvent varies with temperature whereas the mass of a solvent does not. Therefore osmolarity measurements are temperature dependent, while osmolality is temperature independent.

> **REMEMBER** !
>
> One osmole equals one mole of solute particles. This can be applied as shown by equation 1.5.

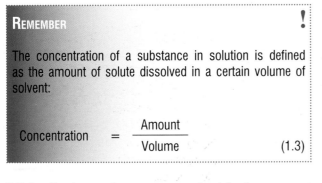

$$\text{Osmolal concentration} = \text{Molar concentration} \times \text{Number of dissociable particles} \qquad (1.5)$$

This can be adapted to calculate osmolarity (Osm/L), as exemplified by the equation below:

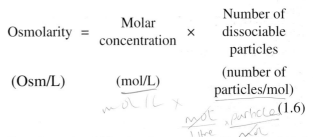

$$\underset{\text{(Osm/L)}}{\text{Osmolarity}} = \underset{\text{(mol/L)}}{\text{Molar concentration}} \times \underset{\substack{\text{(number of} \\ \text{particles/mol)}}}{\text{Number of dissociable particles}} \qquad (1.6)$$

Therefore, the following is true regarding 1 mole of glucose, a single particle when dissolved, in a 1 litre solution:

- Molarity (molar concentration) = 1 mol/L
- Osmolarity = 1 Osm/L.

However 1 mole of a substance that dissociates into 2 solute particles on dissolving in 1 litre of solution (e.g. NaCl) has:

- Molarity (molar concentration) = 1 mol/L
- Osmolarity = 2 Osm/L.

This concept is illustrated in Figure 1.2.

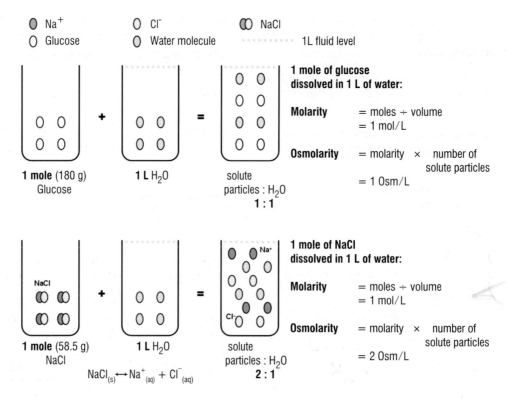

Figure 1.2 – Comparison of molarity and osmolarity

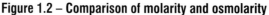

> **REMEMBER** !
>
> **Isosmotic** solutions have the same osmolarity (i.e. equal solution concentrations).
>
> Solutions with a higher or lower osmolarity (e.g. relative to the normal ECF) are termed **hyperosmotic** and **hyposmotic** respectively.

POINTS OF INTEREST 1.2

The concentration of solutes that tend to dissociate on dissolving in a solvent is expressed in terms of 'equivalence'.

Fluid exchange

Hydrostatic pressure and osmotic pressure

> **REMEMBER** !
>
> **Osmosis** describes the net diffusion of water across a selectively permeable membrane, down its concentration gradient i.e. from a region of higher water concentration, across the cell membrane to a region of lower water concentration.

Hydrostatic pressure is the pressure exerted by a stationary fluid on a membrane. As water passively diffuses across the membrane by osmosis:

- It predominantly enters one compartment
- Its presence increases the fluid volume and raises the hydrostatic pressure in that compartment, pushing water out (Fig.1.3).

Hydrostatic pressure is one of the Starling forces which influence filtration across the membrane (see Ch. 4).

The **osmotic pressure** of a solution reflects the tendency for water to passively move into that solution, down its (water) concentration gradient i.e. the tendency for osmosis to occur in the direction of the solution in question.

> **REMEMBER** !
>
> The water concentration gradient is determined by the relative concentration of non-penetrating (impermeant) solutes and water, in each fluid compartment.

The relationship between the three terms defined above (osmosis, hydrostatic pressure and osmotic pressure) can be considered as follows:

- Osmosis is driven by the osmotic pressure of a solution, which depends on the concentration gradient across the cell membrane.
- Osmosis will occur as long as this concentration gradient is maintained, due to the osmotic pressure.

- As osmosis moves more water from one fluid compartment into another, the hydrostatic pressure builds in the compartment being 'filled'.

- Hydrostatic pressure acts to push water in the opposite direction to that of osmosis driven by the osmotic pressure.

- Osmosis stops when the hydrostatic pressure exactly counter-balances the osmotic pressure.

Therefore, the osmotic pressure is equal to the hydrostatic pressure, which is the precise amount of pressure required to prevent osmosis.

Tonicity

The **tonicity** of a solution is its effect on the volume of a cell bathed in the solution. The effect a solution has on a

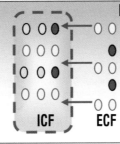
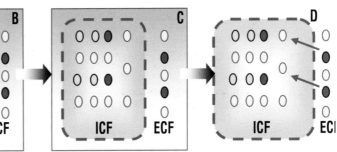

O Impermeant intracellular solute particle
● Permeant extracellular solute particle (e.g. urea solution)
O Water molecule

- - - Cell plasma membrane
⟶ Movement of water by osmosis
⟶ Movement of permeant solute particles

Figure 1.3 – Effect of hypotonic solution on a cell

	ICF	ECF	Solution OSMOLARITY (relative to cell)	Net movement
A	total solute : water 2 : 3	permeant solute : water 2 : 3	ISOSMOTIC	Cell is bathed in a **hypotonic** and **isosmotic** solution of **permeant solute** **ICF [water] = ECF [water]** No net movement of water across the cell membrane **ECF [solute] > ICF [solute]** Permeant solute particles diffuse down their concentration gradient to enter the cell.
B	1 : 1 1 : 3	1 : 3	HYPOSMOTIC	**ECF [solute] = ICF [solute]** No net movement of solute particles across the cell membrane **ECF [water] > ICF [water]** Water moves down its concentration gradient to enter the cell.
C	2 : 3	2 : 3	ISOSMOTIC	**ICF [water] = ECF [water]** No net movement of water across the cell membrane
D	2 : 9	2 : 3		**ECF [solute] > ICF [solute]** Extracellular permeant solute particles diffuse down their concentration gradient to enter the cell **This again creates an osmotic gradient and thus more water moves into the cell by osmosis, causing the cell to swell and eventually burst.**

Note that the solution remains hypotonic (relative to the cell) throughout.
The **tonicity** of a solution depends on **impermeant solute** concentration.

cell's volume depends on the solution's concentration of impermeant solutes relative to the cell's concentration of impermeant solutes. If there is a difference in this concentration across the cell membrane, osmotic pressure drives the passive movement of water into or out of the cell, via osmosis.

An **isotonic** solution has a concentration of impermeant solutes equal to that of the cell, and so does not cause a change in cell volume.

When a cell is bathed in a **hypotonic** solution, there is a lower concentration of impermeant solutes extracellularly, compared with the higher intracellular concentration of impermeant solutes. This means there is a higher water concentration in the extracellular compartment, so osmotic pressure will drive the passive diffusion of water down its concentration gradient into the cell by osmosis. Therefore the intracellular volume increases and the cell swells.

A **hypertonic** solution has a higher concentration of impermeant solutes than that of the intracellular compartment. Bathing cells in a hypertonic solution causes the cells to shrink because water leaves the cells by osmosis to enter the hypertonic environment. Thus, the intracellular volume decreases.

> **REMEMBER** !
>
> In contrast to tonicity, the terms used to describe the osmolarity of a solution (isosmotic, hyposmotic and hyperosmotic) do not indicate whether or not the solute can permeate the cell membrane.

When given the osmolal concentration (osmolarity or osmolality) of a solution, the permeability of the membrane to the solute concerned must be considered. An isosmotic solution of impermeant solute is isotonic, having no effect on the volume of the cells it surrounds. In comparison, an isosmotic solution of permeant solute can behave as a hypotonic solution, causing cells to swell (Fig. 1.3). An important example of a permeant solute is urea, which freely traverses the red blood cell membrane via specific uniporters. Sucrose is an example of an impermeant solute that cannot cross the plasma membrane.

Plasma-colloid osmotic (oncotic) pressure

The term **oncotic pressure** refers to the magnitude of the osmotic pressure exerted by large molecules in solution, which drives the movement of fluid across capillary membranes. Plasma proteins are of particular significance, so oncotic pressure is commonly referred to as **plasma-colloid osmotic pressure.** The normal oncotic pressure generated by plasma proteins is approximately 26–28 mmHg.

Plasma-colloid osmotic pressure is one of the Starling forces that influence filtration across the membrane (see Ch. 4).

> **REMEMBER** !
>
> The balance between the plasma-colloid osmotic (oncotic) pressure and hydrostatic pressure determines the distribution of ECF between the plasma and interstitial fluid.

KEY POINTS 1.2

Molarity refers to the concentration of a substance dissolved in a solution.

Osmolal concentration (expressed as osmolarity or osmolality) is calculated by the multiplication of molar concentration (molarity) by the number of solute particles:

- **Osmolarity** – total number of solute particles (osmoles) in a **litre of solvent** (Osm/L)

- **Osmolality** – total number of solute particles (osmoles) in a **kilogram of solvent** (Osm/kg).

1 osmole = 1 mole of solute particles.

Tonicity is the effect of a solution on cell volume:

- **Isotonic** solutions do not change the volume of a cell

- **Hypotonic** solutions cause cells to swell

- **Hypertonic** solutions cause cells to shrink.

The relationship between a solution's tonicity and the volume of a cell can easily be appreciated by simply remembering two statements along with the definition of osmosis:

1. Tonicity refers to the effect of the extracellular solution on cell volume

2. Tonicity depends on the impermeant solute concentration of the extracellular fluid (the solution) compared to that of the intracellular fluid (impermeant solute concentration inside the cell)

3. Osmosis is the net movement of water across the cell membrane, from a region of high water concentration to a region of low water concentration.

CLINICAL RELEVANCE 1.3 ✚

REMEMBER !

The primary aim of rehydration therapy is to replace any body fluid losses, both in terms of volume and composition (e.g. replacing plasma losses with plasma in burns cases, infusing whole blood to treat acute haemorrhage, and oral rehydration therapy for diarrhoeal losses).

Where oral rehydration is not a suitable option, different types of **replacement fluids** can be administered intravenously, to target the compartment that is volume depleted. The distribution of water depends on the relative effects of the administered solution, on the different body fluid compartments. The appropriate replacement fluid is chosen accordingly.

Replacement fluid products can be broadly categorised:

Crystalloid solutions

- e.g. Specified volume of water as 5% dextrose – distributes equally into all body fluid compartments

- e.g. Specified volume of water as 0.9% saline (NaCl) – isotonic, so stays in the ECF (mainly interstitial)

- Crystalloids may be hypotonic, isotonic or hypertonic

Colloid solutions

- e.g. albumin, fresh frozen plasma, starch products

- Remains in the plasma (vascular compartment of the ECF)

- Colloids are termed 'plasma expanders'.

ASK YOURSELF 1.2 ?

Oral water and sodium salts
5% dextrose infusion
0.9% saline infusion
Colloid solution

Q1. Which treatment from the above list is the most appropriate choice for mild or chronic extracellular volume depletion (e.g. due to excessive renal losses)?

Q2. Which treatment from the above list is the correct choice for hypovolaemia (decreased circulating volume) and why?

Q3. Why is water administered intravenously as 5% dextrose and not as pure water?

A1. Oral water and sodium salts.

If oral rehydration is not possible, an infusion of 0.9% saline is the correct treatment for extracellular water depletion.

A2. Colloid solution has a high oncotic pressure, so it stays in the vascular compartment of the ECF.

A3. Pure water is hypotonic relative to plasma. An infusion of pure water would cause osmotic lysis of blood cells (see *Key points 1.2*).

REGULATION OF BODY FLUID BALANCE

The cell membrane that divides the ICF and ECF is highly permeable to water but not to most electrolytes. Thus water is able to move freely and quickly between these different body fluid compartments. The distribution of fluid across these two major fluid compartments depends on the osmotic effects exerted by Na^+ and Cl^-, and to a lesser extent, the other electrolytes.

In contrast, the ECF compartments (plasma and interstitial fluid) are divided by the capillary membrane which is highly permeable to small ions. The movement of water between the plasma and interstitial fluid relies on plasma-colloid osmotic pressure as well as another force – hydrostatic pressure.

The maintenance of body fluid balance relies on the regulation of two factors, governed by NaCl and water balance:

- ECF volume

- ECF osmolarity.

Na^+ (with its major attendant anions Cl^- and HCO_3^-) is a key determinant of ECF volume and ECF osmolarity. That said, changes in Na^+ balance affect ECF volume, but not its osmolarity; Na^+ imbalances should not alter ECF Na^+ concentration under normal circumstances because of the action of the anti-diuretic hormone (ADH) and thirst systems described below. H_2O balance is a major determinant of ECF osmolarity. Disorders of H_2O balance manifest as changes in plasma osmolarity, and thus abnormal plasma $[Na^+]$.

ECF volume and NaCl balance

> **REMEMBER** !
>
> Na^+ is the major cation in the ECF, along with its attendant anions (Cl^- and HCO_3^- being most significant).

Na^+ salts account for the majority (> 90%) of the ECF's osmotic activity. Changes in ECF salts are accompanied by corresponding changes in ECF water, so control of salt balance is crucial for the maintenance of ECF volume. This requires a salt input that is equal to salt output.

Mechanisms for regulating salt input are limited to **ingestion**. Dietary salt consumption typically exceeds the body's daily requirement. Salt output, in contrast, relies on three routes by which salt is excreted from the body:

- **Perspiration** – minor obligatory loss

- **Faeces** – minor obligatory loss

- **Urinary excretion** – major mechanism (accounting for ~90% of salt output) under the precise control of the kidneys.

> **REMEMBER** !
>
> Sodium is:
> - Freely filtered at the glomerulus
> - Actively reabsorbed
> - Not secreted by the tubule.

Thus the following can be said about renal handling of Na^+:

$$Na^+ \text{ excreted} = Na^+ \text{ filtered} - Na^+ \text{ reabsorbed}$$

(see Ch. 5)

The kidneys respond to deviations in ECF volume associated with changes in the salt load (i.e. the total quantity of salt) via two processes:

- primarily by a hormonal mechanism altering Na^+ reabsorption in the renal tubule (Renin-Angiotensin-Aldosterone system)

- reflex adjustment in glomerular filtration rate (GFR).

Mechanisms for the regulation of ECF volume and blood pressure are described in Chapter 4.

Renal retention of salt is usually accompanied by the conservation of H_2O, which may osmotically follow Na^+ reabsorption. This means that the kidneys conserve an isotonic salt solution. Renal excretion of NaCl and water is regulated by changes in:

- Plasma (vascular) volume
- Blood pressure
- Cardiac output.

These variables are primarily detected by sensors situated in large blood vessels. The coupling of these sensors to the kidneys occurs by neural and hormonal signalling. Sensors of ECF volume and plasma [Na^+] are also found in the liver and central nervous system, but these sensors appear to play a less significant role compared with vascular sensors.

The kidneys are capable of excreting Na^+ over a wide range of concentrations, as required to handle variations in Na^+ input, whilst maintaining a relatively stable ECF volume and Na^+ load in the body. This renal compensatory response occurs over a period of hours to days. So in a case of acute change in salt intake, during the delay there is an imbalance in Na^+. If Na^+ input exceeds its output, there is a **positive Na^+ balance**, while an excess Na^+ output relative to Na^+ input, results in a **negative Na^+ balance**.

Signalling systems involved in regulating renal excretion of both NaCl and H_2O can be categorised as shown in Table 1.4.

Table 1.4 – The effects of signals involved in the control of renal NaCl and water excretion

Signal	Effect of signal activation
Neuronal Renal sympathetic nerves	↓ NaCl excretion
Renin-Angiotensin-Aldosterone system	↓ NaCl excretion
Natriuretic peptides Atrial natriuretic peptide, Brain natriuretic peptide, Urodilatin	↑ NaCl excretion
Anti-diuretic hormone	↓ H_2O excretion

Renal sympathetic nerves

Sympathetic nerve activity is stimulated in response to a negative Na⁺ balance, sensed by baroreceptors (see *Points of interest 1.3*). Adrenergic innervation of the kidneys acts in three ways, described in Table 1.5. Its main effects are:

- Constriction of afferent and efferent arterioles of the glomerulus

- Secretion of renin

- Direct effects on NaCl handling.

Renin-Angiotensin-Aldosterone system

Na⁺ reabsorption is also governed by the Renin-Angiotensin-Aldosterone system. This potent regulatory system responds to changes in:

- NaCl

- ECF volume

- Arterial blood pressure.

In the face of decreased ECF volume, the Renin-Angiotensin-Aldosterone system acts to conserve Na⁺ by promoting Na⁺ reabsorption in the proximal tubule, distal tubule and collecting duct. Na⁺ retention is followed osmotically by H_2O retention, raising ECF volume and elevating blood pressure back toward normal. In response to a rise in arterial blood pressure, the activity of the Renin-Angiotensin-Aldosterone system is appropriately reduced. The role of the Renin-Angiotensin-Aldosterone system in disease states is described in *Clinical relevance 1.5*.

In the blood, renin serves as a proteolytic enzyme acting to cleave angiotensinogen, a plasma protein that is synthesised in the liver and circulates at high levels in the blood as the pro-peptide for angiotensin I. While passing through the pulmonary circulation, angiotensin I (a 10-amino acid peptide) undergoes cleavage by angiotensin converting enzyme (ACE), releasing angiotensin II (an 8-amino acid peptide). This series of reactions is depicted as a continuous pathway in Figure 1.4.

Activation of this system relies on kidney secretion of renin, which occurs by the stimulation of granular cells of the juxtaglomerular apparatus (see Ch. 4). Specific indications for this are a decline in NaCl, ECF volume or blood pressure. The three factors responsible for stimulating renin secretion are outlined below:

1. Perfusion pressure –
   Granular cells and afferent arterioles together function as intra-renal high-pressure baroreceptors, stimulating renin secretion in response to a fall in blood pressure.

2. Sympathetic nerve activity –
   Sympathetic innervation of granular cells and the afferent arteriole is mediated by β-adrenoceptors, and stimulates renin secretion in response to a fall in blood pressure. This is a baroreceptor reflex.

Table 1.5 – Renal sympathetic nerve activity in response to negative Na⁺ balance

Stimulated process	Effects of renal sympathetic innervation	
	Receptors involved	Response
Afferent and efferent arteriole constriction	α-adrenoceptors	Disproportionate vasoconstriction: Afferent arteriole > Efferent arteriole ↓ Hydrostatic pressure in glomerular capillary ↓ GFR ↓ Filtered load of Na⁺
Renin secretion	β-adrenoceptors	Acts as part of Renin-Angiotensin-Aldosterone system, promoting: ↑ Angiotensin II ↑ Aldosterone ↓ Na⁺ excretion
NaCl reabsorption	α-adrenoceptors	Major effect on proximal tubule Na⁺ reabsorption ↑ Body load of Na⁺

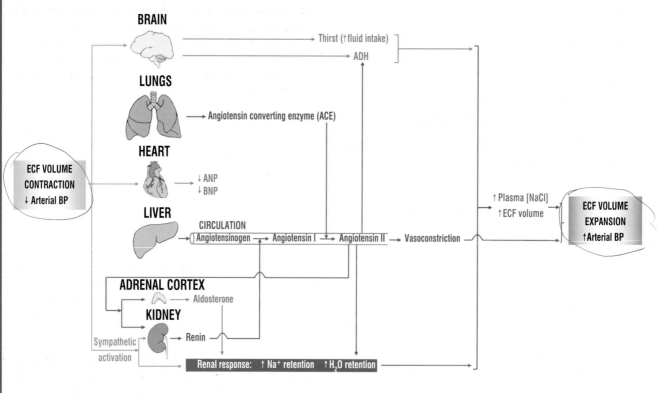

Figure 1.4 – Overview of the Renin-Angiotensin-Aldosterone system and inter-related mechanisms for body fluid regulation

3. Delivery of NaCl to the macula densa – Macula densa cells of the juxtaglomerular apparatus stimulate granular cells in response to a decrease in NaCl in the tubular fluid.

The main functions of angiotensin II are:

*   stimulating the adrenal cortex to secrete the hormone aldosterone

*   stimulating constriction of systemic arterioles

*   stimulating ADH secretion and thirst

*   promoting NaCl reabsorption along the nephron (directly at the proximal tubule and via aldosterone at more distal segments).

Angiotensin II mediates vasoconstriction of the efferent arteriole at the glomerulus, important in regulating blood flow and GFR (see Ch. 4).

Aldosterone is a steroid hormone synthesised in the glomerulosa cells of the adrenal cortex (see Ch. 3). The two primary stimuli for aldosterone secretion are:

*   Angiotensin II

*   ↑ Plasma [K⁺].

The cellular actions of aldosterone that promote Na⁺ reabsorption are described in Chapter 5, including mechanisms increasing Na⁺ transport into cells across the luminal (apical) membrane and Na⁺ transport into the blood across the basolateral membrane.

Natriuretic peptides

Natriuretic peptides promote vasodilatation and induce urinary excretion of Na⁺ and water, so this Na⁺-losing system generally acts in opposition to the Renin-Angiotensin-Aldosterone system.

Myocytes in the heart produce and store atrial natriuretic peptide (ANP) and brain natriuretic peptide (BNP), both of which are secreted in response to dilatation of the heart, as occurs with ECF volume expansion. The kidneys produce a chemically similar natriuretic peptide called urodilatin which only induces NaCl excretion by the kidneys.

As a signalling system in the control of renal NaCl and water excretion, natriuretic peptides have the following effects:

- ↑ GFR

- ↓ Renin secretion

- ↓ Aldosterone secretion (indirectly via inhibition of angiotensin II and directly by inhibiting aldosterone production in the adrenal glands)

- ↓ Reabsorption of NaCl and water by the collecting duct

- ↓ ADH secretion and inhibition of ADH action on the distal tubule and collecting duct.

Nephrotic syndrome is a pathological state in which this system dysfunctions (see *Clinical relevance 1.4* and Ch. 4).

CLINICAL RELEVANCE 1.4 ✚

In **nephrotic syndrome** sodium accumulates in the ECF due to failure of the natriuretic peptide control mechanism. Increased catabolism of cyclic guanosine monophosphate (cGMP), a second messenger that ANP signalling is reliant on, results in unopposed renal retention of sodium. This electrolyte imbalance along with other contributing factors (e.g. release of pro-inflammatory substances that indirectly increase capillary permeability) results in fluid retention with development of oedema.

The pathophysiology and clinical manifestations of nephrotic syndrome are described in Chapter 4.

POINTS OF INTEREST 1.3 💭

Volume sensors located in the circulatory system are known as baroreceptors because they detect and respond to the stretching of the walls of the receptor, induced by changes in blood pressure. The vascular baroreceptors are well understood and can be grouped according to their location within the vascular system:

Low-pressure baroreceptors
- Cardiac atria
- Right ventricle
- Large pulmonary vessels.

High-pressure baroreceptors (arterial side of circulation)
- Aortic arch
- Carotid sinus
- Arterioles of the kidneys.

CLINICAL RELEVANCE 1.5 ✚

Abnormalities of Renin-Angiotensin-Aldosterone system activation can impair renal regulation of Na⁺ and water, with

pathological consequences. Adrenal cortex disease can result in elevated levels of aldosterone **(hyperaldosteronism)** with wide ranging effects including increased Na⁺ reabsorption (mainly in the distal tubule and collecting duct) and reduced urinary excretion of NaCl. This has the following consequences:

- ↑ ECF volume

- ↓ Sympathetic tone

- ↓ Renin, ↓ Angiotensin II

- ↓ ADH

- ↑ ANP, ↑ BNP

Thus, this can be responsible for some cases of hypertension, and can exacerbate congestive cardiac failure by fluid retention and oedema. A deficiency of aldosterone **(hypoaldosteronism)** has the opposite effects with the body in a state of negative Na⁺ balance, resulting in plasma volume contraction.

Other effects of excess aldosterone can be explained by considering the physiology of the renal tubular system, which is described in detail in Chapter 5:

- Aldosterone acts to promote tubular secretion of K⁺ in exchange for Na⁺ reabsorption in principal cells of renal collecting tubules, resulting in hypokalaemia and muscle weakness in individuals with hyperaldosteronism.

- Aldosterone causes H⁺ secretion in exchange for Na⁺ reabsorption in the intercalated cells of cortical collecting tubules, resulting in mild alkalosis in people with hyperaldosteronism

Pathological causes of abnormal aldosterone levels are described in *Clinical relevance 1.9.*

KEY POINTS 1.3 ♪

Body intake of salt is determined by its ingestion.

Output of body salt occurs mainly in urine (perspiration and faeces make minor contributions).

Adjustments in renal tubule handling of water and solutes enable maintenance of body fluid volume and osmolality.

Renal excretion of NaCl and water is influenced by the following signals:

- Neuronal

- Renin-Angiotensin-Aldosterone system

- Natriuretic peptides

- ADH.

1

Sympathetic (adrenergic) innervation of the kidneys, in response to a fall in ECF volume, stimulates three processes:

1. Afferent and efferent arteriolar vasoconstriction
2. Renin secretion
3. NaCl reabsorption.

The following factors stimulate renin secretion from granular cells:

- ↓ Perfusion pressure
- ↑ Sympathetic nerve activity
- ↓ NaCl delivery to the macula densa.

Activation of the Renin-Angiotensin-Aldosterone system is dependent on renin secretion and occurs via proteolytic cleavage of circulating peptides:

$$\text{Angiotensinogen} \xrightarrow{\text{Renin}} \text{Angiotensin I} \xrightarrow{\text{ACE}} \text{Angiotensin II}$$

The steroid hormone aldosterone is produced by the adrenal cortex in response to:

- Angiotensin II
- ↑ plasma [K$^+$].

Angiotensin II and aldosterone act to promote Na$^+$ reabsorption along the nephron, to restore ECF volume in response to hypovolaemia.

CLINICAL RELEVANCE 1.6 ✚

The ratio of body water:sodium may be abnormally decreased or increased, causing abnormalities in serum [Na$^+$]:

- **Hyponatraemia** – serum [Na$^+$] < 135 mmol/L (one of the most commonly encountered electrolyte imbalances)

- **Hypernatraemia** – serum [Na$^+$] > 145 mmol/L (much rarer than hyponatraemia and usually due to water deficit).

Hyponatraemia

Causes –

- **Hyponatraemia with normal ECF volume (abnormalities in ADH activity)**

  Drug-induced ↑ ADH sensitivity

  Abnormal ADH release

  - Severe hypokalaemia (see *Clinical relevance 1.8*)

  - Adrenocortical insufficiency as in Addison's disease (see *Clinical relevance 1.9*)

ADH-like and ADH-stimulating substances e.g. mannitol stimulates osmotic ADH release (see Ch. 5)

SIADH (see *Clinical relevance 1.7*)

- **Hyponatraemia with ↑ ECF volume**

  Cardiac failure and liver failure with cirrhosis

  Iatrogenic e.g. hypotonic fluid administration → hyposmotic expansion (see *Key points 1.2*)

- **Hyponatraemia with ↓ ECF volume**

  Renal losses

  Osmotic diuresis

  Iatrogenic (e.g. excessive diuretic use)

  Adrenocortical insufficiency as in Addison's disease (see *Clinical relevance 1.9*)

  Tubulointerstitial nephritis (see Ch. 5)

  Extra-renal losses

  Gastrointestinal (vomiting, diarrhoea, haemorrhage)

  Skin (perspiration, burns trauma)

  Transcellular (third space) losses

Clinical consequences –

Features of severe hypernatraemia (serum [Na$^+$] > 150 mmol/L) are mostly neurological:

- Headache
- Nausea and vomiting
- Lethargy
- Irritability
- Diminished tendon reflexes
- CNS depression
- Seizures.

Acute hyponatraemic encephalopathy may occur, which constitutes a medical emergency.

Hypernatraemia

Common causes –

- **Excessive sodium intake**

  Iatrogenic e.g. hypertonic intravenous fluid administration (see *Key points 1.2*)

  Hyperaldosteronism (see *Clinical relevance 1.5*)

  Salt poisoning

- **Excessive water excretion**

  ADH deficiency e.g. central diabetes insipidus

Insensitivity to ADH e.g. nephrogenic diabetes insipidus (see Ch. 5)

Osmotic diuresis e.g. hyperosmolar non-ketotic coma (particularly affects patients with type 2 diabetes mellitus)

- **Deficient water intake**

Clinical consequences –
Although the features of hypernatraemia are often non-specific, convulsions may result from severe hypernatraemia.

Key clinical signs and symptoms:
- Dehydration
  - Prolonged capillary refill time (>2 s)
  - ↓ Skin turgor
  - Dry mucous membranes

- Hypernatraemic dehydration
  - 'Doughy' skin
  - Irritability/confusion
  - Weakness/lethargy.

Clinical assessment of hydration and fluid requirements can be challenging, but should be carried out promptly and accurately. Fluid replacement that is too rapid can have fatal consequences including the development of cerebral oedema and 'coning' (brain stem herniation). Fluid requirements can be calculated based on body mass-dependent values for the 24 h maintenance requirement and for the fluid deficit. The type of fluid replacement product to be administered is chosen according to the clinical situation (see *Clinical relevance 1.3*)

Water balance

> **REMEMBER** !
>
> Control of free H_2O balance is critical in order to maintain a stable ECF osmolarity.

If the body's water balance is to be maintained, water input must equal water output exactly. On a daily basis, almost equal amounts of water are typically added to the body by drinking liquids and consuming food. H_2O is also produced metabolically. In clinical situations an important therapeutic route of water entry is intravenous infusion of fluid (see *Clinical relevance 1.3*). H_2O output may be due to:

- Insensible water loss (of which we are normally unaware)
- Sensible water loss.

Sensible water losses occur through:
- Perspiration – varies with physical activity, environmental temperature and humidity, and certain pathological states

- The gastrointestinal tract – only a small amount of water is normally lost through faeces, but gastrointestinal water loss can increase with diarrhoea or vomiting.

Examples of **insensible H_2O losses** include:
- Pulmonary expiration of air moistened in the respiratory passages

- Evaporation of water through skin cells, even in the absence of perspiration (this tends to be limited by the external keratinised dermal layer, but if the skin is significantly damaged as can occur with burn injuries, this waterproofing effect may be impaired resulting in excessive insensible water loss via this avenue).

The final and most important mechanism of water output is **urinary excretion**, which is precisely controlled by renal mechanisms for dilution and concentration of urine (see Ch. 5). When water input exceeds its output, the body experiences a positive water balance and the kidneys respond by producing a high volume of urine that is hyposmotic (relative to plasma). In contrast, when a negative water balance occurs the kidneys produce a small volume of hyperosmotic urine.

> **REMEMBER** !
>
> The ability to vary the osmolality of excreted urine over a wide range (50–1400 mOsm/kg H_2O) allows regulation of water excretion to occur independently of the regulation of solute excretion.

Two major mechanisms regulate renal H_2O excretion:
- Anti-diuretic hormone (ADH)
- Thirst system.

Anti-diuretic hormone

ADH, also known as vasopressin, is a 9-amino acid peptide produced in neuroendocrine cells situated in the supraoptic and paraventricular nuclei of the hypothalamus. Synthesised ADH is then transported to the posterior pituitary gland for storage prior to its release. ADH secretion is dependent on the following factors, denoted as stimulatory (+) or inhibitory (−):

Major factors:

(+) ↑ Effective osmolality of body fluids (sensed by osmoreceptor cells in the anterior hypothalamus)

(+) ↓ Pressure of the vascular system (sensed by low- and high-pressure baroreceptors located in the circulatory system).

Other factors:

(+) Nausea

(+) Angiotensin II

(−) Atrial natriuretic peptide.

Inappropriate factors (unrelated to the body's H_2O balance):

(+) Stress-related factors e.g. pain, fear

(−) Alcohol.

Of these factors, osmotic and haemodynamic control are the most potent. ADH is rapidly synthesised and degraded in response to minor deviations in plasma osmolality and blood volume or pressure, making this a highly sensitive system. The role of ADH in renal physiology is described in Chapter 5.

ADH primarily acts to increase:

- Water permeability of the collecting duct

- Urea permeability along the inner medullary collecting duct.

Posterior pituitary syndromes involving ADH are described in *Clinical relevance 1.9* and Chapter 5.

CLINICAL RELEVANCE 1.7 ✚

The **syndrome of inappropriate ADH secretion (SIADH)** is caused by conditions that alter the normal nervous stimulation of ADH secretory cells (e.g. intracranial infections and neoplasms, pulmonary diseases, certain drugs).

SIADH is characterised by:

- Excess circulating ADH levels

- Overexpression of water channels in the collecting duct of the renal tubule (see Ch. 5)

- ↑ Water reabsorption (water retention results in hypo-osmotic body fluids).

Thus the major clinical manifestations include hyponatraemia and cerebral oedema.

Thirst system

The thirst centre is a neural centre situated in the same region as the hypothalamic control centre that regulates ADH secretion. Generally, ADH secretion and thirst are activated simultaneously and work in concert:

- actively conserving body water (by the actions of ADH on the kidneys)

- stimulating thirst (the sensation that triggers water intake).

Thus, the control of ADH secretion and thirst depends on some similar factors:

- ECF osmolality

- ECF volume or blood pressure.

Other thirst-stimulating factors are angiotensin II secretion and a dry mouth.

The most powerful stimulus for thirst is **hypertonicity** – even minor elevations in plasma osmolarity trigger a relatively strong desire to drink. Immediate relief of thirst upon drinking is transient and complete satisfaction of thirst is only achieved when plasma osmolality or blood volume or pressure are restored to normal and no longer stimulating the thirst system.

Potassium balance

REMEMBER !

K^+ is the major cation in the ICF, along with its attendant anions (PO_4^{3-} and negatively charged proteins trapped within cells).

The majority (98%) of the body's K^+ is located intracellularly. ECF $[K^+]$ is normally maintained at about 4.2 mmol/L by precise control mechanisms. **Hyperkalaemia** occurs at an ECF $[K^+] > 5.0$ mmol/L while an ECF $[K^+] < 3.5$ mmol/L constitutes **hypokalaemia**. Disturbances of K^+ balance (common causes and how they manifest) are described in *Clinical relevance 1.8*.

CLINICAL RELEVANCE 1.8 ✚

Hyperkalaemia

A serum $[K^+] > 6.0$ mmol/L usually requires urgent treatment.

Common causes –

- Impaired excretion of potassium

  - Renal failure
  - Drug-induced, including dietary potassium supplements, ACE inhibitors, K^+-sparing diuretics (see Ch. 5), heparin, non-steroidal anti-inflammatory drugs (NSAIDs) like aspirin
  - Hypoaldosteronism e.g. Addison's disease (see *Clinical relevance 1.9*)

- Enhanced cellular release of potassium

  - Acidosis
  - Diabetic ketoacidosis (see*Clinical relevance 1.9*)
  - Rhabdomyolysis (or tissue damage)
  - Spurious causes.

Clinical consequences –

If the rise in extracellular potassium ion concentration is severe enough, it constitutes a medical emergency progressively leading to cardiac toxicity, development of arrhythmia and eventually cardiac failure. arrest

Hyperkalaemia is commonly associated with metabolic acidosis, with specific respiratory effects described in Chapter 2.

Hypokalaemia

Defined as serum $[K^+] < 3.4$ mmol/L.

Common causes –

- Increased renal excretion of potassium

  - Drug-induced, with thiazides, loop diuretics and osmotic diuretics (see Appendix 1)

- Hyperaldosteronism

  - Liver failure
  - Cardiac failure
  - Nephrotic syndrome (see Ch. 4)
  - Cushing's syndrome (hypercortisolaemia either due to exogenous corticosteroid therapy or of endogenous origin e.g. ACTH-producing tumours)
  - Conn's syndrome (see *Clinical relevance 1.9*)

- Gastrointestinal losses e.g. vomiting.

Amongst the other causes of hypokalaemia, is renal tubular disease (see Ch. 2).

Clinical consequences –

Although hypokalaemia is usually asymptomatic, muscle weakness or constipation may result from severe hypokalaemia. Interstitial renal disease is associated with chronic hypokalaemia.

It is important to be aware that hypokalaemia predisposes an individual to toxicity from digoxin, a cardiac glycoside drug used to increase myocardial contraction, sometimes indicated in the treatment of heart failure and some specific types of arrhythmia.

Regulation of ECF [K⁺]

Major factors influencing K^+ distribution between the ECF and ICF are:

- Hormonal (physiological) control (Fig. 1.5)
- Pathophysiological factors altering plasma $[K^+]$

Hormonal (physiological) control –

Hormones released in response to a rise in plasma $[K^+]$, act to increase K^+ uptake into body tissues by stimulating transporters in skeletal muscle, liver, bone and red blood cells:

- Adrenaline

- Insulin

- Aldosterone.

K^+ uptake can be increased acutely by the up-regulation of preformed transporters – Na^+/K^+-ATPase pump, $Na^+/K^+/2Cl^-$ symporter and Na^+/Cl^- symporter. Alternatively, K^+ uptake can be increased over a period of hours to days by increasing the number of Na^+/K^+-ATPase transporters in responsive cells.

Secretion of catecholamines (adrenaline in particular) activates ß-adrenoceptors, causing K^+ uptake from the ECF into cells. The importance of these hormone actions on K^+ distribution, in terms of normal human physiology and their dysfunction in pathological states, is considered in *Clinical relevance 1.9*.

Pathophysiological factors that alter plasma $[K^+]$ –
- Acid-base balance:

  The effects of H^+ concentration on the movement of K^+ between the ICF and ECF are partly attributed to H^+-inhibition of Na^+/K^+-ATPase activity. Metabolic acidosis causes an increase in ECF $[K^+]$ whereas metabolic alkalosis results in a fall in ECF $[K^+]$.

- Cell lysis:

  The destruction of cells results in release of their contents (K^+ and other intracellular solutes) into the ECF, so

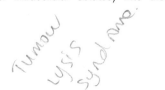
Tumour lysis syndrome

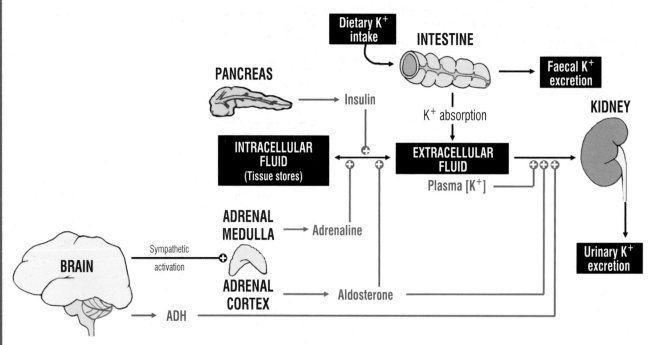

Figure 1.5 – Overview of K⁺ homeostasis

extensive tissue injury can cause severe hyperkalaemia. Important examples include burn injuries, rhabdomyolysis (destruction of skeletal muscle) and lysis of red blood cells (as occurs in haemolytic anaemia and gastric ulcer bleeding resulting in digestion of blood cells).

• Exercise:

Especially strenuous or prolonged exercise causes significant K⁺ release from skeletal muscle cells into the ECF, normally resulting in mild, self-limiting hyperkalaemia. However this may cause symptoms in some individuals who lack the necessary compensatory mechanisms e.g. patients with endocrine disorders, renal failure or taking certain medications like ß-blockers.

• Plasma osmolarity:

A rise in ECF osmolarity causes water to leave cells osmotically. In patients with diabetes mellitus, high plasma glucose concentration causes a rise in ECF osmolarity and cellular dehydration, which promotes movement of K⁺ out of cells, increasing ECF [K⁺]. Conversely, decreased plasma osmolarity has the opposite effect.

• Drug-related (see *Clinical relevance 1.8*)

Two important examples of drugs that increase plasma [K⁺] include ACE inhibitors and K⁺-sparing diuretics. The mechanism of action of K⁺-sparing diuretics is described in Chapter 5.

CLINICAL RELEVANCE 1.9

Outlined below are examples of hormonal control of K⁺ distribution between the ECF and ICF, and how this is altered in disease states:

> **REMEMBER** !
>
> Stimulation of all three hormones (adrenaline, insulin and aldosterone) promotes K⁺ uptake by responsive cells (Fig. 1.5).

Adrenaline –
Following exercise, intracellular K⁺ is released from skeletal muscle. ß-adrenoceptor stimulation is important in preventing exercise-induced hyperkalaemia. Hypokalaemia is a potential adverse side effect of ß₂-agonists.

Insulin –
Insulin is the major stimulatory hormone for movement of extracellular K⁺ into cells post-prandially i.e. after a meal. In patients with **diabetes mellitus (DM)** the actions of insulin are diminished (due to insulin deficiency in type 1 DM and impaired insulin sensitivity in type 2 DM) therefore the post-prandial rise in ECF [K⁺] is greater than normal. Insulin and glucose administered intravenously help correct severe hyperkalaemia in emergencies.

Aldosterone –
Addison's disease is characterised by adrenal insufficiency and aldosterone deficiency, associated with clinically significant hyperkalaemia (high ECF [K⁺] due to the lack of aldosterone-induced K⁺ uptake into cells and insufficient aldosterone-induced renal K⁺ excretion). Common causes of the adrenal cortex destruction that underlies Addison's disease, include autoimmune disease and tuberculosis. Characteristic features of Addison's disease include postural hypotension, progressive weakness, loss of appetite, weight loss and skin hyperpigmentation (see *Points of interest 1.4*).

Patients with **Conn's syndrome** have increased aldosterone secretion (primary hyperaldosteronism) resulting in hypokalaemia, hypertension and muscle weakness. This relatively rare condition is usually caused by a benign tumour of the adrenal cortex, or excessive growth of the adrenal glands (see Ch. 3).

It should be noted that aldosterone is controlled by plasma [K$^+$] and angiotensin II. Figure 1.4 provides an overview of the Renin-Angiotensin-Aldosterone system.

POINTS OF INTEREST 1.4

In Addison's disease, the primary problem of non-responsiveness of the adrenal gland to ACTH, results in mineralocorticoid deficiency. Thus the normal negative feedback from mineralocorticoids (inhibiting ACTH synthesis) is lost. Metabolism of the ACTH precursor hormone stimulates melanocytes, causing hyperpigmentation of the skin, oral mucosa and gums.

KEY POINTS 1.4

K$^+$ balance is maintained in the body primarily by regulation of renal K$^+$ excretion to match dietary K$^+$ intake i.e. input = output.

Many cell functions are sensitive to ECF [K$^+$] so mechanisms are also present to maintain ECF [K$^+$] following gastrointestinal absorption into the ECF after a meal.

Only 5–10% of K$^+$ intake is lost through perspiration and faeces.

REMEMBER !

Renal K$^+$ excretion in urine is the primary mechanism involved in potassium homeostasis, responsible for excreting 90–95% of dietary K$^+$ intake.

Therefore advanced renal disease renders the kidneys unable to eliminate K$^+$ from the body, resulting in hyperkalaemia (see *Clinical relevance 1.8*). Cellular mechanisms of K$^+$ secretion by principal cells in the distal tubule and collecting duct are described in Chapter 3 and 5.

K$^+$ excretion by the kidneys depends on the **rate** of three processes:
1. Potassium filtration at the glomerulus (GFR × plasma [K$^+$])
2. Reabsorption of potassium into the blood
3. Secretion of potassium into the tubule.

K$^+$ is free (unbound) in the plasma and so it is freely filtered at the glomerulus.

Major factors influencing K$^+$ secretion are:
- Physiological factors that regulate K$^+$ balance
  - Plasma [K$^+$]
  - Aldosterone
  - ADH (less significant role).
- Pathophysiological factors that disturb K$^+$ balance
  - Tubular fluid flow rate – Increases with diuretic treatment and ECF volume expansion, and rapidly promotes K$^+$ secretion.
  - Acid-base balance – Extracellular [H$^+$] affects Na$^+$/K$^+$-ATPase activity and the permeability of the luminal membrane to K$^+$. Metabolic acidosis (high plasma [H$^+$]) reduces K$^+$ secretion by these mechanisms, while alkalosis has the opposite actions.
- Glucocorticoids – Increase excretion of K$^+$ in the urine. The mechanisms involved are described in *Points of interest 1.5*.

POINTS OF INTEREST 1.5

Glucocorticoids increase urinary K$^+$ excretion via two mechanisms:
1. Increasing GFR which increases tubular flow rate
2. Stimulating the activity of an aldosterone-induced protein kinase that mediates trafficking of epithelial Na$^+$-selective channels to the cell membrane. This mechanism involves the serum- and glucocorticoid-regulated kinase gene (*Sgk1*).

KEY POINTS 1.5

The regulation of body fluid balance is dependent on control of ECF volume and ECF osmolarity.

The renal system provides the major route for tightly regulated excretion of water and NaCl.

ECF volume is monitored by multiple sensors. The primary sensors, known as volume receptors or baroreceptors (pressure-sensitive), are located in the large vessels of the vascular system.

The Renin-Angiotensin-Aldosterone system is a key regulator of the body's salt balance, promoting salt conservation during urine formation (with osmotic water retention).

The stimulation of renin is dependent on three factors:
1. Perfusion pressure
2. Sympathetic nerve activity
3. Delivery of NaCl to the macula densa (see Ch. 4).

Key regulators of the body's water balance are:

- ADH (vasopressin) – regulates kidney water retention during urine formation

- Thirst system – triggers desire to drink.

Both ADH secretion and thirst are stimulated by changes in:

- Effective plasma osmolality

- Blood pressure

- ECF volume

- Angiotensin II.

Secretion of the hormones adrenaline, insulin and aldosterone promotes K^+ uptake into body cells.

The primary site for regulating K^+ excretion is the principal cell of the late distal tubule and cortical portion of the collecting duct (see Ch. 5).

INTEGRATIVE CASE STUDY

AD is a 44-year-old female of Asian origin, currently living in the UK. AD sees her physician complaining of easy fatigability and loss of appetite. During the past month she has lost 6 kg. She has a previous history of tuberculosis.

On examination, AD appears clinically dehydrated, has marked hyperpigmentation of the skin and postural hypotension, with her blood pressure falling upon assuming an upright posture (110/65 mmHg supine and 80/55 mmHg erect).

Blood test results:

Plasma [Na$^+$]	= 130 mmol/L	[135 – 145 mmol/L]
Plasma [K$^+$]	= 6.0 mmol/L	[3.5 – 5.0 mmol/L]
Plasma [HCO$_3^-$]	= 20 mmol/L	[22 – 28 mmol/L]
Plasma [glucose]	= 2.8 mmol/L	[3.5 – 7.8 mmol/L] random glucose

Diagnosis?

- This is likely to be **Addison's disease** (primary chronic adrenocortical insufficiency due to destruction of the adrenal cortex).

- Important features:

  - Non-specific – progressive **weakness**, easy **fatigability**, gastrointestinal disturbances (e.g. anorexia, nausea, vomiting, **weight loss**)
  - ↑ Plasma [ACTH precursor hormone] → melanocyte stimulation → hyperpigmentation
  - In some cases, ↓ glucocorticoids → hypoglycaemia (glucocorticoids have a role in normal glucose metabolism e.g. opposing insulin)

- Characteristic fluid and electrolyte disturbances due to ↓ mineralocorticoid (aldosterone) activity, particularly important in solute handling in the late distal tubule and collecting duct (see Ch. 5) –

  - Hyperkalaemia: ↓ K^+ secretion by P cells → ↑ plasma [K^+]
  - Hyponatraemia: ↓ Na^+ reabsorption by P cells → ↓ plasma [Na^+]
  - Hypotension: Negative Na^+ balance → ↓ plasma volume → ↓ BP
  - Metabolic acidosis: ↓ H^+ secretion by IC cells → ↓ HCO_3^- reabsorption → ↓ plasma [HCO_3^-]

Other causes and features of metabolic acidosis are described in Chapter 2.

Aetiology?

- The majority of cases of Addison's disease are due to:

  - Autoimmune adrenalitis (accounts for 60–70% of all cases)
  - Tuberculosis (given this patient's past medical history, tuberculous disease may be the underlying cause)
  - Acquired Immune Deficiency Syndrome (AIDS) and HIV infection
  - Metastatic cancers.

- There are many other possible aetiologies e.g. lymphomas, amyloidosis (see Ch. 4), fungal infections.

- Generally, Addison's disease can affect people of any race and either gender (but autoimmune causes are much commoner in Caucasian women).

- Conditions that may be associated with Addison's disease include autoimmune thyroid disorders.

Further investigations?

In addition to the serum electrolytes and blood glucose (see above) the following investigations may be necessary:

- Full blood count (FBC)
  - white blood cell profile may be abnormal
- Short ACTH test
  - Synthetic ACTH (Synacthen) is given to stimulate adrenal cortisol production.
- ACTH and cortisol levels

- Adrenal autoantibodies

- Chest X-ray for tuberculosis

- Imaging of adrenal glands (e.g. abdominal X-ray for calcification).

Management?

- Management depends on the underlying aetiology.

- Patients with autoimmune Addison's disease require lifelong regular steroid replacement therapy e.g. prednisolone.

- In the UK and USA, this patient would be advised to carry a steroid card and wear a Medic Alert bracelet (to communicate details of the wearer's medical conditions to others, in case of Addisonian crisis when emergency replacement therapy may be required in a confused or unconscious patient).

Self-Assessment

Questions:

Body fluid distribution

1. Are the following statements regarding body fluid compartments **true or false**?

   (a) The two major divisions of body fluid, the intracellular and extracellular fluid compartments, are separated by the capillary endothelial wall. F
   (b) A healthy adult weighing ~70 kg will have a total body water of ~60 L. F
   (c) Extracellular concentration of sodium (135–145 mmol/L) normally exceeds its intracellular concentration (9 mmol/L). T

2. Are the following statements regarding the body fluid status of a patient (55-year-old male) with congestive heart failure **true or false**?

Blood test results:	Plasma [Na$^+$] = 130 mmol/L [135 – 145 mmol/L] — Plasma [K$^+$] = 2.8 mmol/L [3.5 – 5.0 mmol/L] ↓
Examination findings:	Distended neck veins Pulmonary oedema and pitting ankle oedema Pulse rate = 120 beats/min Blood pressure = 100/70

   (a) The presence of oedema indicates an increase in the extracellular fluid volume. T
   (b) The electrolyte disturbances are compatible with a positive water balance. F ✗ —
   (c) The electrolyte disturbances are compatible with increased urinary excretion of K$^+$. T

General principles of fluid balance

3. Are the following statements regarding the placement of red blood cells in different solutions **true or false**?

   Osmolarity of intracellular fluid is 282 mOsm/L (1 osmole = 1000 milliosmoles)
   0.9% solution of sodium chloride is isotonic
   5% glucose solution is isotonic

   Osmolality of intracellular fluid is approximately 300 mOsm/kg H$_2$O
   A 300 mmol/L solution of sucrose is isosmotic (osmolality = 300 mOsm/kg H$_2$O)
   A 300 mmol/L solution of urea is isosmotic (osmolality = 300 mOsm/kg H$_2$O)

   (a) When bathed in a 1.5% solution of sodium chloride the red blood cells will swell. T ✗
   (b) When bathed in a glucose solution of 3% the red blood cells will shrink. F
   (c) When bathed in a 300 mmol/L sucrose solution the volume of the red blood cells remains unchanged. T
   (d) When bathed in an isosmotic solution of urea the volume of the red blood cells remains unchanged. T ✗
   (e) The 300 mmol/L urea solution is isotonic.

Regulation of body fluid balance

4. Are the following statements regarding renal sympathetic innervation **true or false**?

   (a) A fall in ECF volume detected by baroreceptors stimulates sympathetic nerve activity.

(b) Sympathetic innervation of the kidneys causes constriction of afferent and efferent arterioles of the glomerulus via activation of ß-adrenoceptors.

(c) Noradrenergic innervation of the kidneys also stimulates renin release by granular cells and NaCl reabsorption.

5. Are the following statements regarding the Renin-Angiotensin-Aldosterone system **true or false**?

(a) Renin acts as a proteolytic enzyme, cleaving angiotensin I to release angiotensin II.

(b) Aldosterone promotes Na^+ reabsorption in the principal cells and intercalated cells of the collecting duct, in response to hypovolaemia.

(c) Excess production of aldosterone by the adrenal medulla may occur in some pathological conditions associated with excess Na^+ reabsorption and elevated ECF volume that may cause hypertension.

Answers:

(see *Key points 1.1*)
1. (a) False. The ICF and ECF are separated by the cell plasma membrane.
   (b) False. Total body water in an adult is normally 40–45 L, typically accounting for ~60% of body weight.
   (c) True.

(see *Key points 1.3*)
2. (a) True.

> There is a shift in body fluid distribution, with a decrease in the effective circulating volume associated with an increase in ECF volume.

(see *Key points 1.1*)
   (b) True.
   (c) True.

(see *Key points 1.2*)
3. (a) False. The cells will shrink.

> If a solution of 0.9% sodium chloride is isotonic, then sodium chloride solutions of greater than 0.9% are hypertonic. A hypertonic solution causes a decrease in cell volume.

   (b) False. The cells will swell.

> If a glucose solution of 5% is isotonic, then glucose solutions of less than 5% are hypotonic. A hypotonic solution causes an increase in cell volume.

   (c) True. Thus the sucrose solution is isotonic.

> The red cell membrane is impermeable to sucrose, which in a 300 mmol/L solution exerts an osmotic pressure equal and opposite to the osmotic pressure exerted by the intracellular contents (extracellular osmolality = intracellular osmolality). An isosmotic solution of impermeant solute is isotonic. An isotonic solution has no effect on cell volume.

   (d) False. The cells will swell and eventually burst.

> A solute can only exert an osmotic pressure across the plasma membrane if the membrane is impermeable to that solute. Urea easily permeates the red cell membrane, moving down its concentration gradient into cells, and cannot exert an osmotic pressure to counter-balance that exerted by the intracellular contents. Thus its behaves like a hypotonic solution, causing the cell volume to increase.

   (e) False.

> See above, part (d) for explanation.

(see *Key points 1.2*)
4. (a) True. Hence a negative Na^+ balance stimulates sympathetic innervation of the kidneys.

   (b) False. Sympathetic vasoconstriction of the afferent and efferent arterioles is mediated by α_1-adrenoceptors.
   (c) True.

5. (a) False. Renin is the proteolytic enzyme involved in the cleavage of circulating angiotensinogen, the pro-peptide for angiotensin I.

> Angiotensin converting enzyme (ACE) acts in cleaving angiotensin I to release angiotensin II.

(see *Clinical relevance 1.5*)
   (b) True.
   (c) False. Aldosterone is produced in the adrenal cortex.

> The rest of the statement is true – pathological states of hyperaldosteronism are associated with raised ECF volume and some cases of hypertension.

The concentration of unbound (free) hydrogen ions (H^+) in body fluids is under the precise regulation of a number of factors responsible for H^+ secretion. In the human body H^+ concentration ($[H^+]$) is maintained at very low levels relative to the concentration of other ions. Thus the negative logarithm, pH, is employed:

$$pH = -\log[H^+]$$

In general, processes necessary for life are pH-sensitive and cannot occur outside a range of body fluid pH 6.8 – 7.8.

PRINCIPLES OF ACIDS AND BASES

> **REMEMBER** !
>
> Acids are proton donors, whereas bases are proton acceptors.

Dissociation (ionisation)

A strong acid like hydrochloric acid (HCl) has a greater tendency to dissociate (ionise) in solution than a weak acid (e.g. carbonic acid). That is to say upon dissolving in water, a greater proportion of a strong acid's molecules will separate into free H^+ and anions, relative to the proportion of a weak acid's molecules that will dissociate.

The following equations represent ionisation of an acid and a base in water, where:

- A^- is the anion component of an acid (known as its conjugate base)
- B is a basic molecule and BH^+ is its conjugate acid.

The examples show the dissociation of hydrochloric acid and ammonia (reaction with H_2O is implied).

Acid: $\quad \mathbf{HA \leftrightarrow H^+ + A^-} \qquad$ e.g. $HCl \leftrightarrow H^+ + Cl^-$
$\quad$ ($\rightarrow$ favoured at alkaline pH)

$$(2.1)$$

Base: $\quad \mathbf{B + H^+ \leftrightarrow BH^+} \qquad$ e.g. $NH_3 + H^+ \leftrightarrow NH_4^+$
$\quad$ ($\rightarrow$ favoured at acidic pH)

$$(2.2)$$

Chemical buffers

Chemical buffer systems oppose and minimise changes in pH by binding with or yielding, free H^+. A buffer system acts via a reversible reaction between two substances mixed in solution (the buffer pair):

- one acts as an acid (proton donor)
- the other behaves like a base (proton acceptor).

Upon the addition or removal of an acid or base to this solution, the change in $[H^+]$ is opposed by the buffer pair, capable of binding and removing H^+ from solution, or dissociating to release free H^+ into solution.

Henderson-Hasselbalch equation

The relative concentrations of acid and base in a solution determine its pH, while the dissociation constant (K) of an acid or a base specifies its 'strength' in terms of its ability to donate or accept protons respectively. This relationship is expressed as the Henderson-Hasselbalch equation, where $pK = -\log K$:

$$pH = pK + \log \frac{[A^-]}{[HA]} \qquad (2.3)$$

Since the pH of a solution is numerically equal to the pK of an ionised acid or base, the Henderson-Hasselbalch equation is useful for calculating the pH of solutions of weak acids or bases.

How is the Henderson-Hasselbalch equation derived?

> **REMEMBER** !
>
> The abbreviated acid-base reaction (see equation 2.1):
> $HA \leftrightarrow H^+ + A^-$

With the concentration of reactants ([HA]) as the denominator, and the concentration of products ($[H^+][A^-]$) as the numerator, the dissociation constant (K) of an acid reacting with a base (H_2O) is expressed as follows:

$$K = \frac{[H^+][A^-]}{[HA]} \qquad (2.4)$$

Equation 2.4 is rearranged as shown below:

$$[H^+] = K \frac{[HA]}{[A^-]} \qquad (2.5)$$

The Henderson-Hasselbalch equation is derived by taking the negative log of each term (see equation 2.3).

Bearing in mind the three key concepts covered at the beginning of the chapter – dissociation/ionisation, chemical buffer systems and the Henderson-Hasselbalch equation – the function of chemical buffer systems in human physiology can be appreciated. For example, if a strong acid like HCl is added to a buffered solution the acid will dissociate into free H^+ and Cl^- anions. As the $[H^+]$ of the solution begins to rise, the basic member of the buffer pair (B) binds to some of the additional H^+ ions and removes them from the solution thereby minimising the increase in acidity. In a situation of declining $[H^+]$, the acidic member of the buffer pair (AH) dissociates yielding free H^+ which opposes the rising pH. This ability to 'respond' to changes in $[H^+]$ enables body fluids to maintain their pH within the normal physiological range.

REGULATION OF ACID-BASE BALANCE

Normal arterial blood pH is 7.45 and normal venous blood pH is 7.35. So a plasma pH < 7.35 (acidaemia) is considered acidotic, while alkasosis is the term designated to plasma pH > 7.45 (alkalaemia).

In terms of input, humans ingest acidic and alkaline substances. The products of ongoing cellular metabolic activities may be acid or alkali. The main processes that contribute H^+ are:

1. • carbonic acid formation *lactate ketones*

2. • nutrient breakdown producing inorganic acids

3. • intermediary metabolism producing organic acids

4. • additional acids may be produced in certain pathological conditions (see *Clinical relevance 2.3*).

Output of alkali occurs through faecal excretion. The net result of bodily processes (input and output of acid and alkali) is an excess of acid in body fluids. Therefore, the free H^+ generated must be removed from solution within the body and eventually eliminated from the body, in order to maintain the normal alkalinity of the extracellular fluid (ECF) i.e. approximately pH 7.42.

Occasionally conditions may result in excess alkalinity of the ECF. H^+ balance is achieved via three major compensatory mechanisms:

1. Chemical buffer systems
2. Respiratory mechanisms
3. Renal mechanisms

A relatively narrow range of pH 6.8 – 7.8 is compatible with life.

Acidosis occurs at blood plasma pH < 7.35.

Alkalosis occurs at blood plasma pH > 7.45.

Three key compensatory mechanisms are responsible for regulating body acid-base balance:

1. Chemical buffer systems
2. Respiratory mechanisms
3. Renal mechanisms

The three major mechanisms that resist changes in H^+ are described below, in order of the immediacy of their response to fluctuations in pH.

1. Chemical buffer systems – first line response

The body has four buffer systems:

$$CO_2 + H_2O \rightleftharpoons H_2CO_3 \rightleftharpoons H^+ + HCO_3^-$$

1 • Carbonic acid:bicarbonate buffer system
2 • Protein buffer system
3 • Haemoglobin buffer system
4 • Phosphate buffer system.

Each of these systems is important in its own way, and differences in their major functions are summarised in Table 2.1.

Carbonic acid:bicarbonate buffer system

The carbonic acid (H_2CO_3): bicarbonate (HCO_3^-) buffer system is most relevant clinically because it is measurable and because changes in the H_2CO_3:HCO_3^- pair reflect changes in the other buffer systems. This buffer system is unique in that it is regulated both by the kidneys and the lungs:

• Kidneys regulate HCO_3^-

• Respiratory system regulates CO_2.

The other reason the H_2CO_3:HCO_3^- system is such an effective ECF buffer against non-carbonic acid changes, is the abundance of its components H_2CO_3 and HCO_3^- in the ECF. The significance of these components is best understood by considering equation 2.6:

$$\underset{carbonic}{\underset{\rightarrow}{\underset{anhydrase}{CO_2 + H_2O \overset{(slow)}{\leftrightarrow} H_2CO_3 \overset{(fast)}{\leftrightarrow} H^+ + HCO_3^-}}} \quad (2.6)$$

The first reaction of CO_2 hydration/dehydration is normally slow and so it is the rate-limiting step. This reaction is accelerated in the presence of the zinc-containing enzyme carbonic anhydrase, which catalyses the hydration of CO_2 (see *Points of interest 2.2*). The second reaction involving the ionisation of H_2CO_3 to H^+ and HCO_3^- is more immediate.

ASK YOURSELF 2.1 ?

Q. The terms 'acid-forming' or 'H^+-generating' are often used with regard to CO_2, and a rise in CO_2 is frequently related to a rise in [H^+]. Why is this so, when the production of every H^+ from the dissociation of CO_2-generated H_2CO_3 is accompanied by the production of one HCO_3^- ion (see equation 2.6)?

A. Although HCO_3^- is also produced by this reaction, its increase in the plasma is proportionally less compared with the increase in plasma [H^+], which is normally very low. For every single H^+ and HCO_3^- ion produced, the number of H^+ ions doubles from 1 to 2, whereas the number of HCO_3^- ions rises from 600,000 to 600,001.

POINTS OF INTEREST 2.2

The actual reaction catalysed by carbonic anhydrase is:

$$H_2O \rightarrow H^+ + OH^- + CO_2 \rightarrow HCO_3^- + H^+ \rightarrow H_2CO_3$$

The effects on pH of alterations in the buffer pair H_2CO_3 and HCO_3^-, can be determined using the aforementioned Henderson-Hasselbalch equation:

$$pH = pK + \log \frac{[HCO_3^-]}{[H_2CO_3]} \quad (2.7)$$

Alternatively the equation can be expressed in terms of the amount of CO_2 and HCO_3^-. The values necessary to ascertain the amount of CO_2 are the partial pressure of CO_2 (PCO_2) and its solubility (α).

Table 2.1 – Summary of the chemical buffer systems

Chemical buffer system	Primary role
Carbonic acid:bicarbonate buffer system (generated by the hydration of carbon dioxide)	Most important buffer of extracellular fluid against non-carbonic acid changes
Protein buffer system (intracellular protein and plasma protein-based)	Important intracellularly (but also buffers extracellular fluid)
Haemoglobin buffer system (intracellular protein-based)	Buffers H^+ generated from carbonic acid
Phosphate buffer system (tissue component – calcium phosphate in bone)	Important urinary buffer (but also buffers intracellular fluid)

$$pH = pK + \log \frac{HCO_3^-}{\alpha\, PCO_2} \qquad (2.8)$$

The calculated pH can be expressed as $[H^+]$ (see equation 2.9), or $[H^+]$ can be calculated directly from known values for PCO_2 and HCO_3^- concentration (equation 2.10).

$$pH = \log_{10} \frac{1}{[H^+]} \qquad (2.9)$$

$$[H^+] = \frac{24 \times PCO_2}{[HCO_3^-]} \qquad (2.10)$$

Phosphate buffer system

The phosphate system is most significant as a urinary buffer and intracellularly, where phosphates are high in concentration. It is the only body-fluid buffer system that is present to act in the renal tubular system, and depends on renal filtration and excretion of excess phosphate. Thus its buffering role during urine formation is unique.

This system's buffer pair are both phosphate salts:

- one acidic (NaH_2PO_4)
- the other basic (Na_2HPO_4).

These acidic and basic phosphate salts are capable of donating or accepting H^+ respectively (in exchange for Na^+), as and when required to oppose changes in $[H^+]$. The phosphate buffer system is expressed as the following equation:

$$Na_2HPO_4 + H^+ \leftrightarrow NaH_2PO_4 + Na^+ \qquad (2.11)$$

Calcium release also occurs as part of the bone-derived mechanism of extracellular buffering that involves bone demineralisation. This response to acidosis enables removal of H^+ from solution as Ca^{2+}-containing salts bind H^+.

ASK YOURSELF 2.2   **?**

Q. Can you identify four key aspects to be aware of when considering the functions of a chemical buffer system in the human body?

A.

1. **What is its primary role?**

2. **How immediate is the buffering response?**

   Extracellular buffers act virtually instantaneously whereas intracellular buffering occurs more slowly over a period of minutes.

3. **What are the components of the buffer system (the buffer pair) and how are they derived in the body?**

4. **How effective is the buffer system?**

   Often this depends on the concentration of the buffer pair in the relevant body fluid compartment.

By the end of this chapter you should be able to answer all these questions regarding the H_2CO_3:HCO_3^- buffer system and the phosphate buffer system.

REMEMBER   **!**

Some important limitations of chemical buffer systems:

- A buffer system cannot buffer itself

- Buffering simply removes H^+ from solution and does not eliminate H^+ from the body

- Each buffer system has a limited capacity for H^+ exchange and eventually relies on the slower respiratory and renal mechanisms of pH control to eliminate acid from the body.

---

2. Respiratory compensation – second line response

REMEMBER   **!**

The rate of pulmonary ventilation is the rate of gas exchange between the lungs and the atmosphere (O_2 absorption and CO_2 excretion).

CO_2 generates H^+ (see equation 2.6) so excretion of CO_2 from the body essentially lowers $[H^+]$ and raises pH, reducing acidity in body fluids.

PCO_2 is dependent on the rate of ventilation (respiratory rate) and so too is blood pH, due to the relationship between PCO_2 and pH (see equation 2.8). By controlling the rate of CO_2 removal, the respiratory system determines $[H^+]$. An increased rate of respiration (known as hyperventilation) increases the rate of CO_2 removal, reducing blood PCO_2, whereas a decrease in respiratory rate (hypoventilation) results in CO_2 retention and a rise in blood PCO_2. It makes sense then that respiratory rate is governed by blood levels of PCO_2 and H^+, creating a feedback system.

This happens via stimulation of chemoreceptors sensitive to changes in PCO_2 and $[H^+]$. The level of respiratory activity appropriately adjusts, as part of a reflex response involving the stimulation of the respiratory centre in the brain stem (see *Points of interest 2.3*).

POINTS OF INTEREST 2.3

The chemoreceptors involved in sensing the PCO_2 and $[H^+]$ changes that eventually stimulate respiratory compensation, are located centrally and peripherally:

• Central (brainstem) – anterior surface of the medulla oblongata

• Peripheral – carotid and aortic bodies.

REMEMBER !

Hypoventilation acts to raise blood $[H^+]$ by suppressing pulmonary excretion of CO_2. However, a reduced respiratory rate is accompanied by a deficiency of oxygen in body tissues termed hypoxia, which is a potent stimulator of ventilation. This limits the effectiveness of hypoventilation as a compensatory mechanism against metabolic alkalosis.

Other important limitations in the mechanisms responsible for respiratory compensation are listed below:

• Respiratory mechanisms only respond to non-respiratory (i.e. metabolic-induced) imbalances in acid-base balance

• Respiratory mechanisms only partly compensate for metabolic-induced changes in pH.

ASK YOURSELF 2.3 ?

Q. When pulmonary disease is responsible for CO_2 accumulation, which mechanisms contribute to the body's response in restoring a normal pH?

A. When respiratory abnormalities result in altered PCO_2, the change in pH cannot be resolved by respiratory mechanisms. The body then relies on chemical buffer systems other than the H_2CO_3:HCO_3^- system (since a buffer system cannot buffer itself) and renal compensation.

3. Renal (metabolic) compensation – third line response

Despite a delay of a few hours to days, the effects of renal compensation are the most potent in terms of regulating acid-base balance. The kidneys are able to regulate the removal of H^+ and HCO_3^- from the body. This means that renal compensation is much more effective at restoring pH towards normal, compared with respiratory compensation which relies solely on regulation of acid-forming CO_2. Additionally, enzyme-dependent production of ammonium ions (NH_4^+) in the proximal tubule forms part of the response to a pH imbalance; the production and excretion of NH_4^+ can be increased or decreased as required. The time involved in enzyme synthesis and activity accounts for the delay in renal compensation. Table 2.2 summarises the three interrelated renal mechanisms of ion regulation occurring in response to acidosis and alkalosis. These mechanisms are described in further detail below.

Table 2.2 – Summary of renal compensatory mechanisms

Renal Compensation	Acid-base abnormality	
	Acidosis	Alkalosis
Hydrogen ion regulation		
H^+ secretion	↑	↓
H^+ excretion	↑	↓
Bicarbonate ion regulation		
HCO_3^- reabsorption and addition of new HCO_3^- to plasma	↑	↓
HCO_3^- excretion	None (filtered HCO_3^- completely reabsorbed as normal)	↑
Ammonium ion regulation		
(production and excretion of NH_4^+)	↑	↓
Compensatory change in plasma pH		
Blood pH	↑ (alkalinisation towards normal)	↓ (acidification towards normal)

REMEMBER   **!**

Key definitions:

Reabsorption – movement of filtered substances from the tubular lumen back into the vascular compartments surrounding the nephron

Secretion – movement of substances from the vascular compartment into the tubular lumen filtrate

Excretion – movement of filtrate in the tubular lumen out of the body to the external environment.

These processes are illustrated in Chapter 5.

Hydrogen ion regulation

H^+ is continuously generated metabolically, and the persistent addition of acid to body fluids would eventually overwhelm the capacity of chemical buffer systems to remove H^+ from solution. The lungs deal with H^+ derived from carbonic acid, by removing CO_2 through respiration (shifting equation 2.6 to the left). The role of the kidneys is to eliminate excess H^+ derived from other acids e.g. lactic acid.

The kidneys compensate for any systemic acid-base imbalance in two ways:

- Acute response – ↑ transporter activity
- Slower, long-term response – ↑ transporter synthesis.

Both types of response act to up-regulate transporters in the membrane of the nephron. The former response is more immediate and involves altering the number and activity of transporters, while the latter response of increased transporter synthesis requires more time.

REMEMBER   **!**

H^+ filtration rate = plasma $[H^+]$ × GFR   (see Ch. 4)

Plasma $[H^+]$ is normally very low, so an extremely small amount of H^+ is filtered for urinary excretion. The majority of H^+ that is eventually excreted enters the tubular lumen by its active secretion in the proximal, distal and collecting tubules (see Ch. 5).

The effect of plasma pH on renal tubule cells in the nephron is the primary physiological factor influencing the rate of H^+ secretion. A change in the intracellular pH has three key effects (mediated by various hormonal and non-hormonal factors) that influence the rate of cellular H^+ secretion:

- intracellular pH determines the H^+ concentration gradient across the apical (luminal) membrane
- intracellular pH affects the allosteric interactions of transporter proteins
- intracellular pH can stimulate exocytotic membrane insertion of transporters from intracellular vesicles, as occurs in the proximal tubule and intercalated cells of the collecting duct.

Two important mediators of these mechanisms are described in Chapter 4:

- Cortisol – a glucocorticoid hormone produced in the adrenal cortex
- Endothelin – a vasoconstrictor hormone produced by endothelial and proximal tubule cells.

Acidosis stimulates the release of both the hormones cortisol and endothelin, which increase H^+ secretion via their effects on the Na^+/H^+ antiporter and $Na^+/3HCO_3^-$ symporter on the basolateral membrane of the proximal tubule. Alkalosis stimulates the reverse response, thereby enabling renal adaptation.

Secondary factors that regulate H^+ secretion, but not directly related to maintaining acid-base balance, include adjustments in:

- Filtered load of HCO_3^-
- ECF volume
- Angiotensin II
- Aldosterone
- Potassium balance
- Parathyroid hormone (PTH).

The Renin-Angiotensin-Aldosterone system and potassium homeostasis are described in Chapter 1. PTH homeostasis is described in Chapter 5.

Bicarbonate ion regulation

The kidneys regulate plasma $[HCO_3^-]$ in two ways:

- Reabsorption of filtered HCO_3^-
- Addition of new HCO_3^- to plasma.

HCO_3^- is freely filtered at the glomerulus, but the tubule cell's luminal membrane is impermeable to the ion. Therefore, HCO_3^- is reabsorbed in a stepwise manner, as depicted in Figure 2.1 and described below:

1. HCO_3^- reacts with H^+ in the tubular fluid to form H_2CO_3

2. H_2CO_3 is broken down by the action of carbonic anhydrase (CA), to H_2O and CO_2

3. H_2O and CO_2 are reabsorbable and can cross the luminal membrane of the tubule cell

4. Inside the tubule cell, HCO_3^- is formed again from its reactants H_2O and CO_2 (in the presence of intracellular carbonic anhydrase)

5. The basolateral membrane of the tubular cell is permeable to HCO_3^-, so the ion crosses (via Na^+/HCO_3^- co-transporters or HCO_3^-/Cl^- exchangers) and then enters the blood.

6. The Na^+/H^+ antiporter at the luminal membrane permits transport of intracellular H^+ into the tubule lumen, enabling the process of HCO_3^- reabsorption to continue (see point 1).

Thus the entire process of HCO_3^- reabsorption relies on a series of reactions and various transport mechanisms (see Ch. 5).

Normally all the filtered HCO_3^- is reabsorbed because secretion of the H^+ necessary for its conversion to H_2CO_3 in the tubular fluid (and subsequent 'reabsorption'), exceeds the amount of filtered HCO_3^-. The secreted H^+ involved in the process of HCO_3^- 'reabsorption' is not excreted, while the excess secreted H^+ that is not utilised in this way, associates with urinary buffers like basic HPO_4^{2-} for excretion (Fig. 2.2). Any HCO_3^- formed intracellularly by the dissociation of H_2CO_3 produced by cellular metabolic activities, is termed 'new HCO_3^-'. Movement of new HCO_3^- into the plasma is coupled with the excretion of H^+.

Ammonium ion regulation

The buffering capacity of urinary phosphates is exceeded in the presence of high H^+ secretion. So

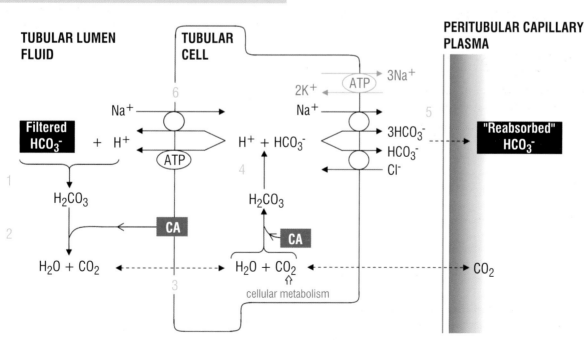

Figure 2.1 – Cellular reabsorption of filtered HCO_3^-

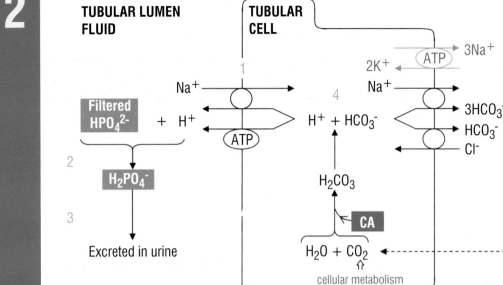

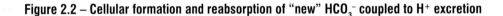

Figure 2.2 – Cellular formation and reabsorption of "new" HCO_3^- coupled to H^+ excretion

1. H^+ leaves the tubule cell via luminal membrane Na^+/H^+ antiporters and H^+-ATPase pumps

2. Secreted H^+ that exceeds the H^+ requirement for processes of HCO_3^- 'reabsorption' (see Fig. 2.1), reacts with filtered HPO_4^{2-} in the tubular fluid to form $H_2PO_4^-$

3. H^+ is eliminated from the body via urinary excretion of $H_2PO_4^-$

4. Inside the tubule cell, HCO_3^- is formed from its reactants H_2O and CO_2, in the presence of intracellular carbonic anhydrase (CA)

5. The basolateral membrane of the tubular cell is permeable to HCO_3^-, so the ion crosses (via Na^+/HCO_3^- co-transporters or HCO_3^-/Cl^- exchangers) and then enters the blood.

renal excretion of H^+ relies heavily on the buffering of secreted urinary H^+ in the collecting tubule, by ammonia (NH_3) produced in the proximal tubule (Fig. 2.2).

REMEMBER !

A titratable acid is a filtered buffer with a conjugate anion (the basic member of the buffer pair) whose concentration range is governed by the physiological pH range of urine. Since the filtered load of a substance is the product of its plasma concentration and GFR (see Ch. 4), titratable acids cannot increase dramatically in acidotic conditions.

Phosphate is the primary titratable urinary buffer.

Following saturation of the urinary phosphate buffer system in acidotic conditions, tubule cells secrete NH_3 into the tubular fluid. NH_3 associates with H^+ in the tubular fluid, forming lipid-insoluble ammonium

(NH_4^+) to which the luminal membrane is poorly permeable (so NH_4^+ tends to remain in the tubular lumen and is excreted). Thus the effect of combining NH_3 with H^+ is two-fold:

- H^+ is 'removed' from the tubular fluid by the incorporation of H^+ into NH_4^+, allowing the kidneys to increase H^+ secretion

- H^+ is eliminated from the body by its excretion in the form of NH_4^+, all in a bid to resist the effects of acidosis.

The reaction involved is: $NH_3 + H^+ \rightarrow NH_4^+$
(see equation 2.2).

POINTS OF INTEREST 2.4

The main source of ammonia is glutamine. The deamination of glutamine to α-ketoglutaric acid and ammonia is catalysed by glutaminase.

ACID-BASE DISORDERS

Acid-base disturbance may be due to respiratory or metabolic causes and the imbalance may be acidotic or alkalotic in nature. Thus deviations from normal acid-base balance are divided into four categories based on the source and direction of the abnormality:

- Respiratory Acidosis
- Respiratory Alkalosis
- Metabolic Acidosis
- Metabolic Alkalosis.

The specific diagnosis is usually determined by the clinical history and examination. Arterial blood gases are measured and specific patterns of change can be detected (see *Clinical relevance 2.5*).

Respiratory acidosis

Causes of respiratory acidosis

Respiratory acidosis is caused by abnormal retention of CO_2 resulting from hypoventilation which may be due to:

- Pulmonary disease
- Depression of the respiratory centre in the brainstem (may be drug-induced e.g. with opioid analgesics like morphine, or caused by disease)
- Neuromuscular disorders that impair respiratory muscle action.

Changes in uncompensated respiratory acidosis

PCO_2 and $[H^+]$ rise.

Compensation for respiratory acidosis

Mechanisms to resist the fall in pH, in order of immediacy of action:

1. Chemical buffer systems bind and remove H^+ from solution.
2. Respiratory compensatory mechanisms are usually ineffective in cases of acid-base disturbance arising from respiratory pathologies.
3. Renal (metabolic) compensation involves retention of HCO_3^- by conserving all filtered HCO_3^- and by adding new HCO_3^-, with concurrent increases in H^+ secretion and excretion (Fig. 2.1 and Fig. 2.2).

Respiratory alkalosis

Causes of respiratory alkalosis

Respiratory alkalosis is caused by increased loss of CO_2 due to hyperventilation which may arise from conditions that stimulate ventilation in an unregulated manner:

- Aspirin toxicity (see *Clinical relevance 2.1*)
- Fever
- Anxiety, pain or fear
- High altitude.

Changes in uncompensated respiratory alkalosis

PCO_2 and $[H^+]$ fall.

Compensation for respiratory alkalosis

Mechanisms acting to lower pH towards normal:

1. Chemical buffer systems release H^+ into solution
2. Since PCO_2 and H^+ normally stimulate ventilation, the fall in PCO_2 and plasma $[H^+]$ resulting from hyperventilation may inhibit ventilation thus hindering the progress of alkalosis (e.g. in the case of fever or anxiety-induced respiratory alkalosis)
3. Renal compensation occurs if alkalosis persists over a period of days. The low $[H^+]$ and low PCO_2 inhibit HCO_3^- reabsorption in the nephron, so the kidneys excrete more HCO_3^-. The kidneys also conserve H^+ in compensation; net acid excretion is reduced since the excretion of titratable acid and NH_4^+ is dependent on high H^+ secretion.

Both respiratory acidosis and respiratory alkalosis have acute and chronic phases, because of the time delay associated with renal compensation.

CLINICAL RELEVANCE 2.1 ✚

The unwanted effects of salicylate drugs like aspirin on acid-base balance are complex, depending largely on the drug dose (Fig. 2.3).

Metabolic acidosis

This is the most common type of acid-base disturbance. Some of the most frequently encountered causes are listed below.

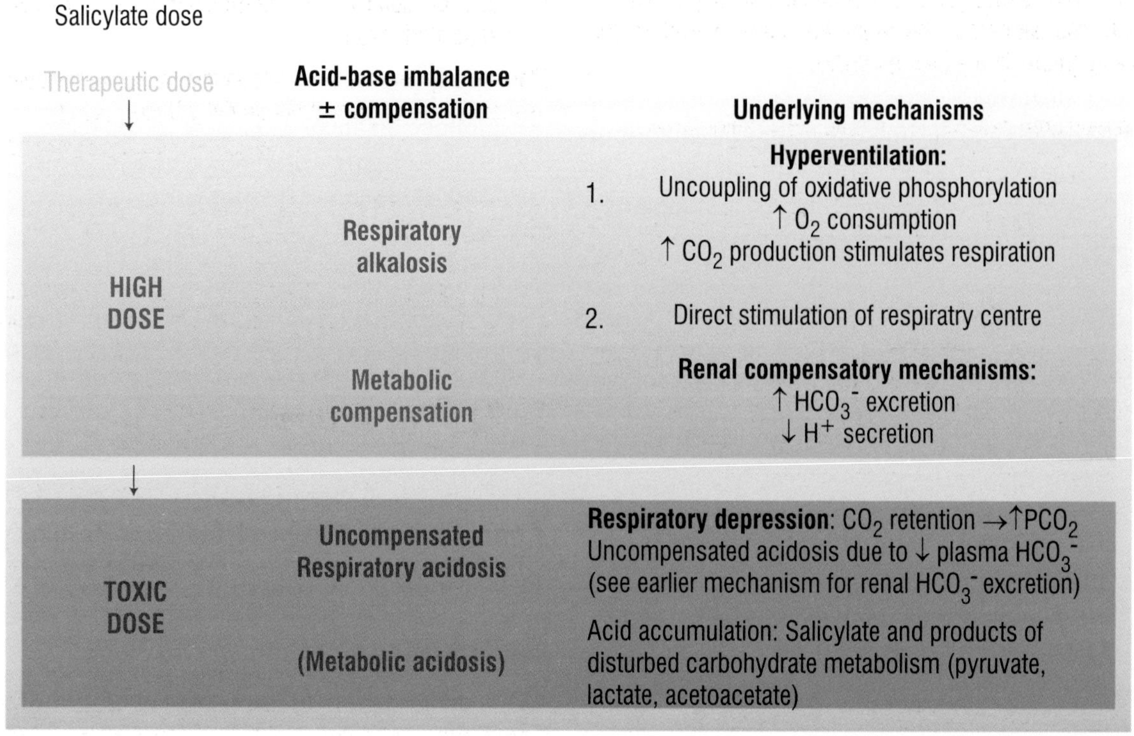

Salicylate dose

Therapeutic dose	Acid-base imbalance ± compensation	Underlying mechanisms
HIGH DOSE	Respiratory alkalosis	**Hyperventilation:** 1. Uncoupling of oxidative phosphorylation $\uparrow O_2$ consumption $\uparrow CO_2$ production stimulates respiration 2. Direct stimulation of respiratry centre
	Metabolic compensation	**Renal compensatory mechanisms:** $\uparrow HCO_3^-$ excretion $\downarrow H^+$ secretion
TOXIC DOSE	Uncompensated Respiratory acidosis	**Respiratory depression**: CO_2 retention $\rightarrow \uparrow PCO_2$ Uncompensated acidosis due to $\downarrow$ plasma HCO_3^- (see earlier mechanism for renal HCO_3^- excretion)
	(Metabolic acidosis)	Acid accumulation: Salicylate and products of disturbed carbohydrate metabolism (pyruvate, lactate, acetoacetate)

Figure 2.3 – Relationship between salicylate dose and adverse effects on acid-base balance

Causes of metabolic acidosis

Metabolic acidosis is caused by the accumulation of any acid except for carbonic acid (which results from excess CO_2 causing respiratory acidosis). Main causes include:

- HCO_3^- losses from the gastrointestinal tract e.g. severe diarrhoea

- Acid generation
  - ketoacidosis due to abnormal fat metabolism in diabetes mellitus (see *Clinical relevance 2.3*)
  - lactic acidosis due to anaerobic glycolysis during strenuous exercise, or as a result of shock or cardiac arrest
- Aspirin toxicity (see *Clinical relevance 2.1*)

- Severe renal failure resulting in uraemic acidosis (uraemic toxicity is due to the accumulation of nitrogenous waste products such as urea in the blood).

Changes in uncompensated metabolic acidosis

Plasma $[HCO_3^-]$ falls and PCO_2 remains unchanged.

Compensation for metabolic acidosis

Uraemic acidosis is the only type of metabolic acidosis that is not compensated for by all three usual mechanisms:

1. Chemical buffer systems bind and remove H^+ from solution.

2. Respiratory centres are stimulated to cause hyperventilation, increasing the excretion of H^+-generating CO_2 (see *Points of interest 2.3*).

3. Retention of HCO_3^- in the kidneys is enhanced by conservation of all filtered HCO_3^- and by the addition of new HCO_3^- (Fig. 2.1 and Fig. 2.2). Net acid excretion increases with increased excretion of titratable acid and NH_4^+.

The excess of H^+ ions in metabolic acidosis causes equation 2.6 to shift to the left. Plasma $[HCO_3^-]$ falls as HCO_3^- ions are used to 'mop up' excess H^+ ions. This hinders the renal compensatory mechanisms described above.

CLINICAL RELEVANCE 2.2 ✚

REMEMBER !

All cations are balanced by anions:

$$[K^+] + [Na^+] + [\text{unmeasured cations}] = [Cl^-] + [HCO_3^-] + [\text{unmeasured anions}] \quad (2.12)$$

Equation 2.13 is rearranged to determine the anion gap, which represents the difference between the unmeasured major cations and anions in the plasma (ECF):

$$[unmeasured\ cations] - [unmeasured\ anions] = ([K^+] + [Na^+]) - ([Cl^-] + [HCO_3^-])$$

$$Anion\ gap = ([K^+] + [Na^+]) - ([Cl^-] + [HCO_3^-]) \quad (2.13)$$

Therefore a change in the anion gap from the normal range (8–16 mmol/L) reflects a change in unmeasured ions. Unmeasured (or unaccounted) anions include phosphate, lactate, keto acids e.g. ß-hydroxybutyrate. Calculating the anion gap can prove useful in determining the cause of a metabolic acidosis:

• *Normal anion gap in acidotic conditions*

- ↑ measured anion e.g. Cl^- in metabolic acidosis due to diarrhoea or renal tubular acidosis
- ↓ HCO_3^- (used to 'mop up' excess H^+) is balanced by ↑ Cl^-
- Anion gap = $([K^+] + [Na^+]) - (↑ [Cl^-] + ↓ [HCO_3^-])$, so no apparent change in anion gap.

• *Increased anion gap in acidotic conditions (i.e. the difference between unmeasured cations and anions increases)*

- ↑ unmeasured anion e.g. in metabolic acidosis due to renal failure, diabetes, lactic acidosis or aspirin overdose
- ↓ HCO_3^- (used to 'mop up' excess H^+) is not balanced by Cl^-, but rather by the unmeasured anion
- ↑ Anion gap = $([K^+] + [Na^+]) - ([Cl^-] + ↓ [HCO_3^-])$.

CLINICAL RELEVANCE 2.3 ✚

Although **diabetic ketoacidosis (DKA)** is a potential complication of either type 1 or type 2 diabetes, DKA affecting the patient with type 1 (insulin-dependent) diabetes, is the more common and more severe scenario. A fall in the insulin:glucagon ratio activates ketogenic processes and metabolic acidosis occurs secondary to the production of several organic keto acids (e.g. ß-hydroxybutyric acid and acetoacetic acid), with a measurable increase in the anion gap (see *Clinical relevance 2.2*).

DKA results in the addition of non-volatile acid to body fluid i.e. acid not derived directly from CO_2 hydration. This has the following effects:

• ↑ plasma $[H^+]$

• ↓ plasma $[HCO_3^-]$, HCO_3^- ions used to 'mop up' excess H^+ ions

• accompanied by ↑ concentration of the non-volatile acid's associated anion.

Plasma hyperosmolarity secondary to hyperglycaemia is associated with hyponatraemic dehydration (see Ch. 1).

POINTS OF INTEREST 2.5

The clinical sign of 'air hunger' (deep, sighing hyperventilation) seen in metabolic acidosis is termed Kussmaul's respiration.

CLINICAL RELEVANCE 2.4 ✚

Renal tubular acidosis (RTA) refers to a spectrum of proximal and distal tubular disorders in which renal net acid excretion is defective, resulting in hyperchloraemic metabolic acidosis, with a normal anion gap (see *Clinical relevance 2.2*).

Proximal RTA (type 2) –

This is due to impaired proximal tubular H^+ secretion and subsequent decreased HCO_3^- reabsorption, associated with generalised tubule dysfunction and reduced activity of transporter proteins. A number of hereditary and acquired conditions are responsible for proximal RTA, including Fanconi's syndrome, cystinosis and nephrotoxin exposure.

HCO_3^- loss is followed by sodium and water. Hypokalaemia usually occurs as a result of increased aldosterone release, in response to plasma volume depletion.

Distal RTA (type 1) –

This occurs when there is a failure of H^+ secretion in the distal tubule and collecting duct. Conditions causing distal RTA may be inherited or acquired. There are both autosomal recessive and autosomal dominant forms of distal RTA, with mutations in the genes encoding specific transporter proteins.

Examples of acquired causes of distal RTA are listed below:

• Medullary sponge kidney – this condition is characterised by multiple cystic dilatations of the medullary collecting ducts

• Drug-induced – the antibiotic amphotericin B alters the H^+ permeability of the distal tubule

• Conditions secondary to urinary obstruction.

Distal RTA may or may not be accompanied by hyperkalaemia, depending on the precise mechanism of disease. In hypokalaemic distal RTA, K^+ is secreted instead of H^+, in exchange for Na^+ reabsorption. In hyperkalaemic distal RTA, voltage defects and hypoaldosteronism impair distal tubular secretion of K^+ and H^+.

Metabolic alkalosis

Metabolic alkalosis is a common cause of acid-base disturbance in hospitalised patients. This is understandable when the causes of metabolic alkalosis are considered e.g. vomiting and diuretic therapy.

Causes of metabolic alkalosis

Metabolic alkalosis is caused by low plasma [H^+] due to a relative deficiency of non-carbonic acids. The causes can be categorised according to the underlying pathophysiology:

- Chloride depletion
    - Gastric losses (vomiting is the most common cause)
    - Diuretics e.g. furosemide
    - Diarrhoea
    - Cystic fibrosis (hereditary disease affecting cells of exocrine glands, with high sweat [Cl^-] being one of its many clinical manifestations)
- Potassium depletion (mineralocorticoid excess) e.g. hyperaldosteronism
- Hypercalcaemia (abnormally high plasma concentration of calcium)
- Ingestion of alkaline drugs
    - Penicillin
    - Bicarbonate ingestion ($NaHCO_3$, baking soda, is a common self-administered antacid therapy).

Changes in uncompensated metabolic alkalosis

Plasma [HCO_3^-] rises and PCO_2 remains unchanged.

Compensation for metabolic alkalosis

Mechanisms act to lower pH towards normal:

1. Chemical buffer systems release H^+ into solution
2. Respiratory centres are inhibited to cause hypoventilation, increasing the retention of H^+-generating CO_2
3. Renal compensation occurs if alkalosis persists for a few days – the low [H^+] inhibits HCO_3^- reabsorption in the nephron, so the kidneys:
    - excrete more HCO_3^-
    - conserve H^+
    - net acid excretion is reduced since the excretion of titratable acid and NH_4^+ is dependent on high H^+ secretion.

KEY POINTS 2.2

Regulation of acid-base balance

Chemical buffer systems:

All chemical buffer systems act immediately, as the first line of defence against acid-base disorders.

Extracellular and intracellular chemical buffer systems form the body's first line of defence against changes in [H^+].

The H_2CO_3:HCO_3^- buffer pair form the:

- principal extracellular fluid buffer system for non-carbonic acids
- only buffer system regulated by both renal and respiratory systems.

The phosphate system is the only buffer system to buffer urine within the tubules of the nephron. Phosphates also play a role in intracellular buffering.

When the body is in a state of acidosis and the phosphate buffer is exhausted, renal tubular cells secrete NH_3, enabling secretion of H^+ to continue and elimination of H^+ by urinary excretion of NH_4^+.

Respiratory compensation:

Respiratory compensation acts at a moderate speed, as the second line of defence against acid-base disorders.

CO_2 is H^+-generating (acid-forming).

Blood levels of PCO_2 and respiratory rate are interdependent.

Chemoreceptors in the brainstem and periphery sense changes in PCO_2 and [H^+] and alter respiratory rate as necessary.

The rate and depth of breathing determine the rate of CO_2 removal:

- Faster and deeper breathing – more CO_2 than usual is "blown off" (excreted)
- Slower and shallower breathing – the rate of CO_2 removal declines and is exceeded by CO_2 production by cellular metabolism (CO_2 accumulates in the blood).

Renal compensation:

Renal mechanisms of pH regulation are the slowest but most powerful, acting as the third line of defence against acid-base disorders.

Renal compensation involves regulation of:

- Hydrogen ions
- Bicarbonate ions
- Ammonium ions.

H^+ secretion depends primarily on the response of tubule cells in the nephron to plasma pH.

HCO_3^- is freely filtered, but its reabsorption occurs indirectly coupled with H^+ secretion, and the regulation of HCO_3^- excretion is dependent on plasma $[H^+]$.

Acid-base disorders

'Respiratory' acid-base disorders are disturbances of acid-base balance resulting from alterations in PCO_2.

'Metabolic' acid-base disorder is the term designated to disturbances of acid-base balance resulting from changes in $[HCO_3^-]$.

Respiratory acidosis:

Common causes: lung disease and depression of respiratory centres.

In response to the high PCO_2 and $[H^+]$:

1. chemical buffer systems remove H^+
2. kidneys retain HCO_3^- (with simultaneous loss of H^+).

Respiratory alkalosis:

Common causes: fever, anxiety and aspirin toxicity.

In response to the low PCO_2 and $[H^+]$:

1. chemical buffer systems liberate H^+
2. respiratory centres may be inhibited, retaining extra CO_2
3. kidneys conserve H^+ and excrete more HCO_3^-.

Metabolic acidosis – the most common type of acid-base disturbance:

Common causes: severe diarrhoea, diabetes mellitus (ketoacidosis) and exercise or cardiogenic shock (lactic acidosis).

In response to the primary decrease in plasma $[HCO_3^-]$:

1. chemical buffer systems remove H^+
2. respiratory centres are stimulated, excreting more CO_2
3. kidneys conserve HCO_3^- and increase net acid secretion.

Metabolic alkalosis

Common causes: vomiting and the use of diuretics (chloride depletion), potassium depletion, hypercalcaemia and drug-induced causes of metabolic acidosis.

In response to the high plasma $[HCO_3^-]$:

1. chemical buffer systems liberate H^+
2. respiratory centres are inhibited, retaining extra CO_2
3. kidneys conserve H^+ and excrete more HCO_3^-.

> **REMEMBER** !
>
> The renal system regulates HCO_3^- while the respiratory system regulates CO_2.
>
> In general terms, acidosis is more worrying than alkalosis and a drop in arterial blood pH must be managed with urgency.

CLINICAL RELEVANCE 2.5 ✚

Normal laboratory values for arterial blood gases (ABGs) are shown below, followed by a table of specific patterns of change seen in different conditions of acid-base imbalance:

Arterial Blood Gases		SI Units
pH	7.35 – 7.45	$[H^+]$ 36 – 44 nmol/L
PCO_2		4.4 – 5.9 kPa
PO_2		10.0 – 14.0 kPa
$[HCO_3^-]$		22 – 28 mmol/L
BE		-2 – +2 mmol/L

BE, Base excess. This is the concentration of base that must be removed in order for pH to return to normal, when PCO_2 is corrected (hence base 'excess'). Thus a negative base excess is sometimes described as a positive base deficit. BE values may be reported alongside or instead of $[HCO_3^-]$.

	pH	PCO$_2$	BE
Respiratory acidosis	Normal or ↓	↑ ↑	↑ (metabolic compensation)
Respiratory alkalosis	Normal or ↑	↓ ↓	↓ (metabolic compensation)
Metabolic acidosis	Normal or ↓	↓ (respiratory compensation)	↓ ↓
Metabolic alkalosis	Normal or ↑	↑ (respiratory compensation)	↑ ↑

Red arrows represent pathological changes, while blue arrows indicate compensatory changes. Therefore, blue arrows in the PCO$_2$ column show respiratory compensation while blue arrows in the BE column reflect metabolic mechanisms of compensation.

INTEGRATIVE CASE STUDY

A 22-year-old male patient, DK, returns home from a tennis tournament and presents to his physician with a 3 day history of worsening nausea and vomiting. DK, a university student, mentions that he has experienced a recent weight loss of about 3 kg over a 3 month period. Apart from mild but recurrent infections of the external genitalia, DK considers himself generally fit and well.

On urinalysis, glucose and ketones are found to be present and a finger-prick test reveals a raised blood glucose. DK is admitted as an emergency case and his condition begins to deteriorate; he appears less alert and has abnormal breathing.

Arterial blood gas results:

pH	=	7.05	[7.35 – 7.45]
PCO$_2$	=	1.60 kPa	[4.4 – 5.9 kPa]
BE	=	-17 mmol/L	[-2 – +2 mmol/L]
PO$_2$	=	14.4 kPa ↑	[10.0 – 14.0 kPa]

ASK YOURSELF 2.2 ?

Using a systematic approach and the normal ABG values provided in grey, interpret the set of ABG results presented in this case. Ask yourself the following questions in a stepwise manner:

1. Is the underlying disorder acidosis or alkalosis? Look at arterial pH

2. Is the acid-base disturbance of respiratory or metabolic origin? Look at PCO$_2$/BE

3. Decide whether compensatory mechanisms are at work. Look at BE/PCO$_2$

4. Is hypoxia present? How does this correlate with the proposed primary process? Look at PO$_2$

Diagnosis?

- This is likely to be a new diagnosis of type 1 diabetes mellitus. Salient features from the history include: nausea and vomiting with or without specific exacerbating factors (e.g. in this case, prolonged period of exercise), weight loss, increased susceptibility to infection.

- The combination of a markedly low pH, low PCO$_2$ and reduced BE indicates a severe primary acid-base disorder of metabolic acidosis, with respiratory compensation. This fits in with the clinical scenario of drowsiness and Kussmaul's breathing (see *Points of interest 2.5*), alongside the results of basic tests which suggest the patient is presenting with diabetic ketoacidosis (see *Clinical relevance 2.3*).

- PO$_2$ is slightly raised, which makes sense since inspired O$_2$ is increased.

Further investigation?

Apart from arterial blood gases, other tests to arrange are listed below and their relevance explained –

- Urea and electrolytes

  - ↑ potassium (typical of this presentation, but levels may be normal)
  - Normal or ↓ sodium levels
  - ↑ urea indicates dehydration

- Laboratory blood glucose

  - This is a more accurate test and should confirm the finger-prick result

- Full blood count (FBC)

  - FBC is a fundamental component of most clinical investigations
  - White cell count may be raised in diabetic ketoacidosis
  - Serum levels of the enzyme pancreatic amylase may be high in diabetic ketoacidosis

- Chest X-ray and electrocardiogram (ECG)

  - These are especially relevant in elderly patients who often have underlying medical conditions

Management?

- The principles of treatment include appropriate management of fluids, insulin and potassium, as well as any general supportive measures that may be necessary. Hypoglycaemia prevents normal inhibition of gastric emptying, so intubation and ventilatory support may be required to prevent aspiration of gastric contents, especially with increasing drowsiness.

- Once the patient is stabilised and becomes well, information and advice should be provided regarding self-monitoring of blood glucose levels, insulin regimens, self-injecting subcutaneous insulin and how to handle episodes of hypo- or hyper-glycaemia, prior to discharge from hospital. A diabetes specialist nurse and dietician will usually be involved in these aspects of long-term management.

- In the UK, this patient is required to notify the Driver and Vehicle Licensing Agency (DVLA) of his health status.

Questions:

Regulation of acid-base balance

1. Are the following statements regarding mechanisms of acid-base balance **true or false**?

   (a) The primary function of the carbonic acid:bicarbonate buffer system is to oppose carbonic acid changes in the extracellular fluid.

   (b) Alterations in levels of PCO_2 and plasma $[H^+]$ stimulate a reflex response in respiratory rate. T

   (c) Under alkalotic conditions, renal tubule cells secrete NH_3. F

   (d) Respiratory centres in the brainstem regulate ventilation primarily in response to centrally located PCO_2-sensitive chemoreceptors. T

Acid-base disorders

2. Are the following statements regarding different clinical situations **true or false**?

   (a) Aspirin poisoning causes metabolic alkalosis due to the effects of salicylic acid. F ✓

   (b) Metabolic acidosis is the most frequently encountered type of acid-base disturbance. T ✓

   (c) Morphine, an opioid analgesic drug, can cause respiratory depression leading to respiratory acidosis. T

3. Are the following statements regarding the acid-base status of a patient with the arterial blood gas results presented **true or false**?

   Arterial blood gas results:

pH	= ↓ 7.22	7.35–7.46 acid acid Resp acid
PCO_2	= ↑ 8.5 kPa	[4.4 – 5.9 kPa]
BE	= -2 mmol/L	[-2 – +2 mmol/L]
PO_2	= ↓ 9.0 kPa hypovent	[10.0 – 14.0 kPa]

   (a) The low plasma pH suggests an underlying disorder of alkalosis. F

   (b) Hypoventilation may be responsible for the rise in PCO_2. T

   (c) The significant fall in base excess probably reflects metabolic compensation in this case.

4.

   Arterial blood gas results:

pH	= ↑ 7.55 alk	Partially comp. Resp alk
PCO_2	= ↓ 3.0 kPa alk	[4.4 – 5.9 kPa]
BE	= ↓ -5 mmol/L acid vent	[-2 – +2 mmol/L]
PO_2	= ↑ 16.0 kPa hyper vent	[10.0 – 14.0 kPa]

   (a) The low PCO_2 suggests a respiratory cause for the alkalosis. T

   (b) There is evidence of metabolic compensation. ✗

   (c) The changes in acid-base balance seen in this set of arterial blood gas results could be due to fever, pain or anxiety.

✓ **Answers:**

(Refer to *Key points 2.2*)

1. (a)   False.
    Remember that a chemical buffer system cannot buffer itself. The H_2CO_3:HCO_3^- system is the primary buffer of extracellular fluid against non-carbonic acid changes.

    (b)   True.
    Adjustments in respiratory activity occur via stimulation of centrally and peripherally located chemoreceptors, sensitive to changes in PCO_2 and $[H^+]$.

    (c)   False.
    Renal tubular secretion of NH_3 occurs when the body is in a state of acidosis and the phosphate buffer is exhausted, enabling further renal secretion of H^+ and H^+ elimination as NH_4^+ excreted in urine.

    (d)   True.

(Refer to *Clinical relevance 2.1*)

2. (a)   False.
    High doses of salicylate drugs can cause initial respiratory alkalosis with metabolic compensation, while toxic doses may result in uncompensated respiratory acidosis plus metabolic acidosis (particularly in children).

(Refer to *Key points 2.2*)

    (b)   True.
    (c)   True.

(Refer to *Clinical relevance 2.5*)

3.   Interpretation of ABG results:

pH < 7.35	↓	acidotic	
PCO_2	↑	respiratory acidosis	
BE		normal	
PO_2	↓	hypoxia	

Since the pH is low, PCO_2 is raised and BE is normal, this is a case of simple respiratory acidosis. Note that the low PO_2 (<10.0 kPa) fits in with a scenario of hypoventilation resulting in CO_2 retention and reduction in inspired O_2.

    (a)   False. Low plasma pH corresponds to acidity.
    (b)   True.
    (c)   False. Base excess is within the normal range.

4.   Interpretation of ABG results:

pH > 7.45	↑	alkalotic	
PCO_2	↓	respiratory alkalosis	
BE	↓	metabolic compensation	
PO_2	↑	hyperoxic	

Since the pH is raised, PCO_2 is low and BE is reduced, this is a case of respiratory alkalosis with metabolic compensation. The rise in PO_2 (> 14.0 kPa) seems logical, since there is suspected hyperventilation.

    (a)   True.
    (b)   True. A decrease in base excess reflects metabolic compensation in a case of respiratory alkalosis.

(Refer to *Key points 2.2*)
    (c)   True.

CHAPTER 3   STRUCTURE OF THE RENAL SYSTEM

Written by: Sandeep Deshmukh, Sunita Deshmukh, Iram Haneef, Newton Wong

GROSS ANATOMY

Kidneys

The kidneys are a pair of reddish brown, 'bean-shaped' organs lying retroperitoneally on the posterior abdominal wall, with one on each side of the vertebral column. They extend from the upper margin of the twelfth thoracic vertebra (T12), down to the level of the third lumbar vertebra (L3), with the right kidney being displaced slightly lower than its left counterpart, presumably due to its close relation to the liver (Fig. 3.2). Each kidney weighs approximately 150 g, and measures around 10–11 cm in length, 6 cm in width and 3 cm in breadth. The left kidney is also recognised to be narrower than the right, may be marginally longer and located closer to the midline, i.e. the vertebral column.

The kidney possesses a 'bean-like' appearance, with a convex lateral surface and concave medial border. Halfway along the medial surface of the kidney is a deep indentation, the renal hilum, which courses into the kidney to communicate with the renal sinus (the space within the kidney). Passing through the renal hilum are the:

- Renal vessels

- Nerves

- Lymphatics (embedded within peri-renal fat).

The structure of the kidney can be divided into two distinct regions – an outer renal **cortex** and an inner renal **medulla** (Fig. 3.1). The outer cortex is covered by the renal **capsule** (thin tissue made up of elastic fibres and collagen) which can normally be easily removed. However, when affected by disease it may adhere to the surface of the kidney.

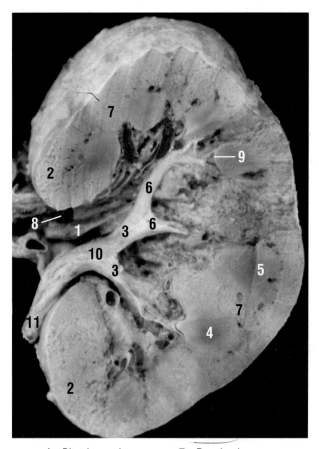

1	Blood vessels	**7**	Renal column
2	Cortex	**8**	Renal hilum
3	Major calyces	**9**	Renal papilla
4	Medulla	**10**	Renal pelvis
5	Medullary pyramid	**11**	Ureter
6	Minor calyces		

Figure 3.1 – Longitudinal section through a kidney showing the internal structure

Renal medulla

The renal medulla lies deep to the cortex and is made up of renal **pyramids**, which possess apices that are directed towards the renal sinus. The renal pyramid bases project outwards and demarcate the junction between the renal medulla and the cortex (i.e. the

Figure 3.2 – Retroperitoneal kidneys and structural relations in the posterior abdominal wall

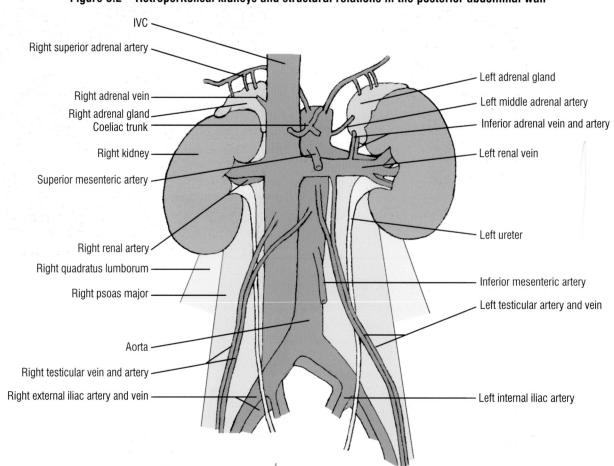

IVC
Right superior adrenal artery
Right adrenal vein
Right adrenal gland
Coeliac trunk
Right kidney
Superior mesenteric artery
Right renal artery
Right quadratus lumborum
Right psoas major
Aorta
Right testicular vein and artery
Right external iliac artery and vein

Left adrenal gland
Left middle adrenal artery
Inferior adrenal vein and artery
Left renal vein
Left ureter
Inferior mesenteric artery
Left testicular artery and vein
Left internal iliac artery

A – Anterior view showing the relationships of ureters, adrenal glands, major blood vessels and muscles

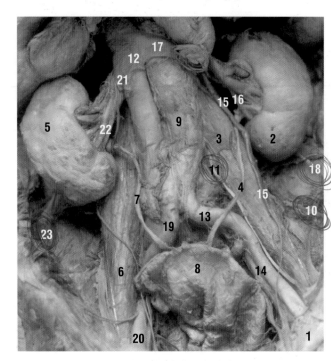

Organs and musculoskeletal structures
1 Inguinal ligament
2 Left kidney (lower pole)
3 Left psoas major
4 Left ureter
5 Right kidney
6 Right psoas major
7 Right ureter
8 Urinary bladder

Vasculature and Innvervation
9 Abdominal aorta and aortic plexus
10 First lumbar spinal nerve
11 Genitofemoral nerve
12 Inferior vena cava
13 Left common iliac artery
14 Left external iliac vessels
15 Left gonadal vein
16 Left renal artery
17 Left renal vein
18 Left subcostal nerve
19 Right common iliac artery
20 Right external iliac artery
21 Right renal vein
22 Right segmental arteries
23 Right subcostal nerve

B – Anterior view dissection

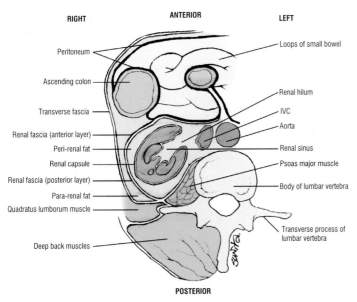

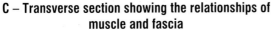

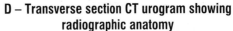

C – Transverse section showing the relationships of muscle and fascia

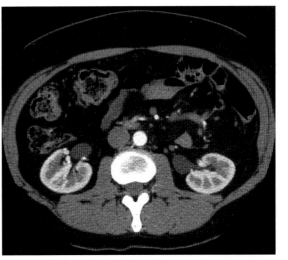

D – Transverse section CT urogram showing radiographic anatomy

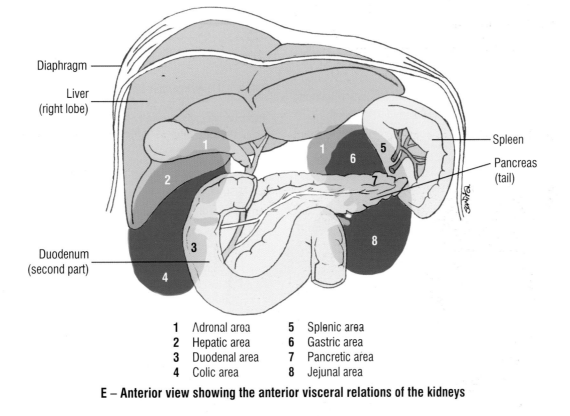

1	Adrenal area	5	Splenic area
2	Hepatic area	6	Gastric area
3	Duodenal area	7	Pancretic area
4	Colic area	8	Jejunal area

E – Anterior view showing the anterior visceral relations of the kidneys

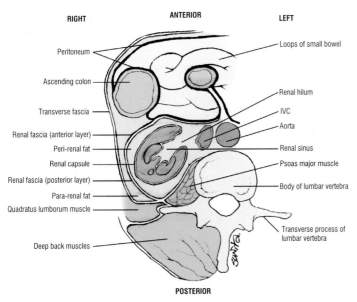

cortico-medullary junction). The pyramid apices form the renal **papillae**, which feed into the **minor calyces**. The minor calyces fuse as they continue towards the renal sinus, into **major calyces**, which fuse to form the renal **pelvis** (situated within the renal sinus). The renal pelvis gives rise to the ureter running vertically downward to enter the bladder.

Renal cortex

The renal cortex can be found between the renal capsule and the bases of the renal pyramids. Cortex intermittently projects in between the renal pyramids, forming renal **columns**.

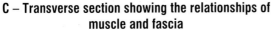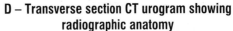

Renal Fascia

The kidneys are encapsulated together with the corresponding adrenal glands by dense connective tissue, the renal fascia. Within the fascia lies adipose tissue (**peri-renal fat**), that completely surrounds the kidney and continues through the **renal hilum** to the **renal sinus**. Its purpose is to act as a shock absorber and to give structural support to the conduit of nerves and vessels which travel through it.

Cystic diseases of the kidney that alter renal morphology are described in *Clinical relevance 3.1*.

CLINICAL RELEVANCE 3.1 ✚

Renal cystic diseases are fairly common. Their aetiology is variable:

- Inherited e.g. polycystic kidney disease
- Acquired e.g. dialysis-associated
- Developmental (non-hereditary) e.g. cystic renal dysplasia.

Sporadic simple cysts are the most common and are almost always asymptomatic with no functional consequence.

Polycystic kidney disease (PKD) is an important genetic form, occurring in about 1 in 800 people. Two distinct patterns of PKD are identified:

- Autosomal dominant PKD (adult)
- Autosomal recessive PKD (childhood).

Autosomal dominant (adult) PKD

- Relatively common
- Major cause of chronic renal failure (see *Clinical relevance 3.2*) usually in fifth decade of life
- Accounts for about 5–10% of all cases of end-stage renal failure requiring transplantation or dialysis

Bilaterally enlarged, multi-cystic kidneys (Fig. 3.3) → Destruction of renal parenchyma → **Renal failure** (typical prognosis)

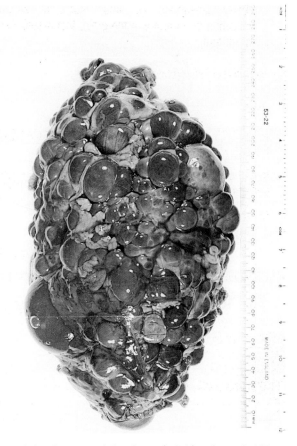

Figure 3.3 – Autosomal dominant (adult) polycystic kidney disease (external surface)
Reprinted with permission from Alan Stevens, James Lowe and Ian Scott. Core pathology, 3rd ed. Mosby, Copyright Elsevier (2008)

The kidney is markedly enlarged and distorted exteriorly with numerous cysts of varying size, between normal renal parenchyma. Hundreds to thousands of cysts may be present, developing from dilated tubules.

- Pathogenesis:
  - Mostly due to mutations in the *PKD1* gene encoding *polycystin-1* protein (up to 90% of cases)
  - Current hypotheses suggest changes in tubular epithelial growth and differentiation associated with abnormalities in the extracellular matrix and epithelial fluid secretion.[9]
- Clinical features:
  - Often asymptomatic initially
  - Flank pain (bleeding and expanding cysts)
  - Haematuria (± blood clot excretion)
  - Mild proteinuria, polyuria, hypertension (and its associated complications) develop progressively
  - Other extra-renal congenital anomalies e.g. hepatic, pancreatic and splenic cysts, heart valve abnormalities
  - *PKD1* encodes proteins in vascular smooth muscle, so another complication of this disease is intracranial

'berry' aneurysm (a small spherical abnormal dilatation of an artery in the brain, that predisposes it to rupture).

Autosomal recessive (childhood) PKD

- Rare

- Majority of cases are perinatal (*in utero*) or neonatal (within the first 28 d after birth)

- It is thought that the pathogenesis involves the *PKHD1* gene that encodes *fibrocystin* protein

- Morphological features:
  - Bilaterally enlarged, externally smooth kidneys
  - Multiple small cysts within renal cortex and medulla

- Congenital liver abnormality (hepatic fibrosis) is an associated clinical feature.

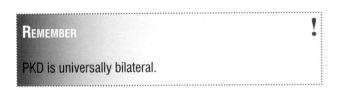

REMEMBER !

PKD is universally bilateral.

Renal vasculature

Arterial supply

The renal arteries arise as lateral branches from the aorta, just inferior to the superior mesenteric artery (Fig. 3.2). Given that the right kidney is further from the midline (and aorta) compared to the left kidney, the right renal artery is also longer and is usually situated higher than the left.

The left renal artery courses behind the left renal vein towards the renal hilum. Along its path it is found posterior to two structures:

- Body of the pancreas

- Splenic vein.

The right renal artery, like the left, courses behind the corresponding renal vein. Along its path the right renal artery is posterior to three structures:

- Inferior vena cava (IVC)

- Descending portion of the duodenum

- Head of the pancreas.

At the renal hilum the renal artery divides into two – an anterior branch and a posterior branch. These continue to branch into five segmental arteries (these are 'end arteries' and therefore do not anastomose). The segmental arteries branch further into lobar arteries, which supply the renal pyramids 1:1 (lobar artery to renal pyramid ratio). Prior to entering the renal parenchyma, the lobar arteries give rise to interlobar arteries which travel alongside the renal pyramids towards the cortex. The interlobar arteries then further divide into arcuate arteries at the cortico-medullary junction. The arcuate arteries project at right angles to the interlobar arteries and give rise to the interlobular arteries coursing throughout the cortex towards the renal capsule (Fig. 3.4).

This flow diagram provides a simplistic overview of the major features of renal vasculature. It is a basic guide to the arterial supply in terms of the sequence of arterial branches.

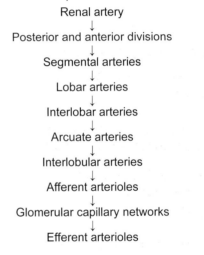

Renal artery
↓
Posterior and anterior divisions
↓
Segmental arteries
↓
Lobar arteries
↓
Interlobar arteries
↓
Arcuate arteries
↓
Interlobular arteries
↓
Afferent arterioles
↓
Glomerular capillary networks
↓
Efferent arterioles

Figure 3.5 – Summary of renal arterial supply

The afferent glomerular arterioles, which form the initial part of the glomerular capillary system, arise mainly from the interlobular arteries (although some do arise from the arcuate arteries). From the glomerular capillary networks the efferent arterioles arise, going on to form the peritubular capillary vasculature around the proximal and distal convoluted tubules. Thus, two sets of capillary networks supply the renal cortex:

- **Glomerular** capillary network – supplies the glomerulus

- **Peritubular** capillary network – supplies the renal tubule.

The situation differs for juxtamedullary glomeruli, with the efferent arterioles from these glomerular tufts going on to form descending vasa recta which supply the medulla (see Ch. 5).

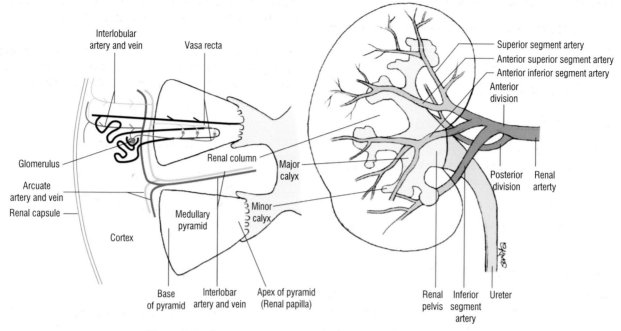

Figure 3.4 – Structural and functional organisation of the kidney

Acute renal failure can be caused by the rapid cessation of blood supply to the kidneys:

- Vascular occlusion

- Central pump failure (cardiac failure → multi-system failure)

- Conditions associated with glomerular, tubular or vascular injury resulting in renal ischaemia, e.g. hypertension, diabetes mellitus, NSAID exposure (see Ch. 4).

Acute renal failure is associated with acute tubular necrosis (see Ch. 5). Other risk factors include:

- Fluid depletion

- Sepsis

- Post-surgery.

At presentation, people in acute renal failure may be **oliguric** (urine output <400 ml/d) and in some instances **anuric** (no urine). This requires timely detection and urgent management.

Chronic renal failure is caused by any condition responsible for progressive nephron loss, including glomerular and tubulointerstitial diseases. Progressive damage to the vasculature of the kidneys resulting in reduced renal blood flow can cause chronic renal failure (e.g. atherosclerosis of the aorta and of the proximal portion of the renal artery). Progressive ischaemic tubular atrophy typically manifests as a gradual decline in glomerular filtration rate (Fig. 3.6).

Amongst the most common causes of end-stage renal failure requiring renal replacement therapy (dialysis or transplantation) are:

- Diabetes mellitus

- Hypertension

- Glomerulonephritis

- Polycystic kidney disease.

The stages described are continuous with one another and there is some degree of overlap.

Stage:		Declining GFR:
1	↓ Renal reserve (asymptomatic)	≥ 90% of normal
2		60–89% of normal
	↓	
3	Renal insufficiency (some clinical features present)	30–59%
	↓	
4	Renal failure (marked metabolic derangement associated with systemic complications)	15–29%
	↓	
5	End-stage renal disease (requires renal replacement therapy e.g. dialysis or transplantation)	< 15%

Figure 3.6 – Chronic renal failure: stages of disease progression

While the injured kidney degrades into a smaller, less (or non-) functional component, the other kidney may undergo hypertrophy to compensate for its deteriorating counterpart.

Chronic complications of declining renal function:

- ↑ **levels of substances normally removed from the body via renal excretion**
- ↓ **production of erythropoietin**
- ↓ **production of vitamin D**

Resulting systemic features:

- **fluid and electrolytes**: usually fluid overload, due to a shift in the normal distribution of body fluid (see Ch. 1), ↑ plasma [K$^+$], metabolic acidosis
- **pulmonary** oedema*
- **cardiovascular**: hypertension, heart failure, pericarditis*
- **gastrointestinal**: nausea and vomiting, bleeding
- **blood disorders** e.g. anaemia
- **bone**: ↑ PO$_4^{3-}$, ↓ Ca^{2+} unless there is hyperparathyroidism secondary to hypocalcaemia (see Ch. 5), bony deformities due to renal osteodystrophy (bone resorption and ↓ mineralisation).
- **neuromuscular** and **dermatological** manifestations.

*pulmonary oedema and pericarditis occur with severe uraemia.

REMEMBER !

Acute renal failure is characterised by a decline in renal function that is rapid and often reversible.

Chronic renal failure implies a more gradual and eventually irreversible deterioration of renal function.

Emergency (acute) problems can occur in both acute and chronic renal failure.

Venous drainage

The veins act as counterparts to the arteries (Fig. 3.4). Beginning at the peritubular plexus, they drain into the interlobular veins and these into the arcuate veins. Further draining into the interlobar and then lobar veins, which course into the segmental and anterior and posterior veins, eventually feeding into the renal veins which ultimately course into the inferior vena cava (Fig. 3.7).

The inferior vena cava is roughly three times longer than the right renal vein (~7.5 cm and ~2.5 cm, respectively). From the renal hilum, the left renal vein courses anterior to the left renal artery and posterior to the body of the pancreas and the splenic vein. The terminal portion of the left renal vein runs anterior to the aorta and into the inferior vena cava (its point of entry into the IVC being slightly superior to that of the right renal vein).

This flow diagram provides a simplistic overview of the major features of renal vasculature. It is a basic guide to the venous drainage in terms of the sequence of venous branches.

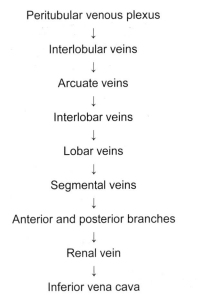

Peritubular venous plexus
↓
Interlobular veins
↓
Arcuate veins
↓
Interlobar veins
↓
Lobar veins
↓
Segmental veins
↓
Anterior and posterior branches
↓
Renal vein
↓
Inferior vena cava

Figure 3.7 – Summary of renal venous drainage

It should be noted that the left gonadal vein (left testicular or ovarian vein) drains into the left renal vein, whereas the right gonadal vein drains directly into the IVC. Due to this, varicocele of the left testicular pampiniform plexus is more common than that of the right plexus.

The right renal vein feeds directly into the inferior vena cava. It travels anterior to the right renal artery and posterior to the descending portion of the duodenum, occasionally crossing behind the lateral portion of the head of the pancreas. Its short length puts it at a higher risk of tearing during renal surgery.

Renal innervation

The kidney is supplied by parasympathetic, sympathetic and visceral afferent fibres from:

- Splanchnic nerves (lower thoracic and upper lumbar)
- Aortic plexus.

Renal lymphatics

The lymphatics can be considered in terms of location:

- Within the renal substance
- Just deep to the renal capsule

Table 3.1 – Comparison of key features of acute and chronic renal failure

	Renal failure	
	Acute	**Chronic**
K+	↑↑	↑
pH	↓ (uncompensated)	↓ (compensated)
Kidney size	Normal/↑	↓
Haemoglobin	Normal unless direct loss or disorder of red blood cells e.g. haemorrhage, haemolysis	↓ even in the absence of bleeding or haemolysis
Bone	Normal	Abnormal

- Within the substance of the peri-renal fat

The glands within the renal substance course along the renal vein towards the **lumbar lymph nodes**, into which they all ultimately drain. The latter two communicate with one another and join the lumbar lymph nodes along the renal vein at the renal hilum.

KEY POINTS 3.1

Gross anatomy: Kidneys

The kidneys are retroperitoneal structures that lie on either side of the midline.
Structural relations:

	Right kidney	Left kidney
Superiorly	Diaphragm (separates kidneys from pleural cavities and 12th pair of ribs)	
Anteriorly		
Superior pole	Right adrenal gland	Left adrenal gland
↓	Liver	Spleen
↓	Duodenum (medial)	Pancreas (medial)
↓	Ascending colon	Descending colon
Inferior pole	Small intestine	Jejunum
Posteriorly	Quadratus lumborum muscle (inferior to diaphragm)	
	Psoas muscle (anteromedial to quadratus lumborum)	

The kidney can be divided into two distinct regions – an outer renal cortex and an inner renal medulla.

The renal pyramids are directed towards the renal sinus. The apex of the renal pyramid (the renal papilla) feeds into a minor calyx. 2–3 minor calyces drain into a major calyx and 2–3 major calyces ultimately into the renal pelvis and down the ureter. This is otherwise known as the collecting system.

Renal pyramid apices (Renal papillae) → Minor calyces → Major calyces → Renal pelvis →Ureter

The kidneys are perfused by the renal arteries, a pair of lateral branches of the aorta.

The right renal artery is longer than the left.

A compromise in the blood supply (acute or chronic) can affect the glomerular filtration rate and integrity of the parenchyma.

The kidneys are ultimately drained by the renal veins, with the right being shorter than the left.

The kidney is innervated by branches of the splanchnic plexus and the aortic plexus.

Three sets of lymph nodes drain into the lumbar nodes.

REMEMBER !

The anatomical planes are:

- **Median** – vertical plane dividing the body into right and left halves
- **Sagittal** – vertical planes parallel to the median plane
- **Coronal (frontal)** – vertical planes perpendicular (at right angles) to the median plane, dividing the body into anterior (front) and posterior (back)
- **Transverse** – horizontal plane perpendicular to the median and coronal planes.

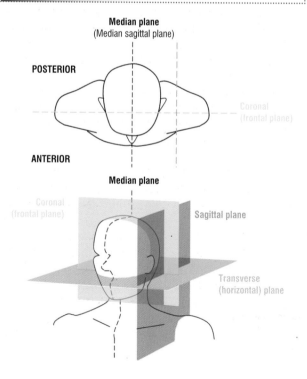

Ureters

The ureters are muscular tubes 25–30 cm in length and ~3 mm in diameter. They are continuous with the renal pelvis and convey urine to the bladder. The thick muscular walls of the ureters generate peristaltic motions to achieve this function.

Figure 3.2 depicts the course of the ureters as they descend the abdominal cavity. Each ureter is normally relatively constricted at three sites. Urinary stones are more likely to arrest at these anatomically narrowed sites (see *Clinical relevance 3.4*). Each ureter begins in the abdomen at the pelvi-ureteric junction, i.e. where the renal pelvis meets the ureter. Each ureter descends slightly medially, its course being retroperitoneal and anteromedial to the psoas major muscle. The ureters effectively lie in the same sagittal plane as the tips of the lumbar vertebral transverse processes, which are located behind psoas major (Fig. 3.9).

At the point of the pelvic brim/inlet, each ureter crosses the bifurcation of the common iliac artery anterior to the sacroiliac joint, to enter the pelvis. Each ureter runs laterally down the pelvic wall, and at the ischial spine turns anteromedially to enter the posterior base of the urinary bladder. Problems associated with the course of the ureters and their insertion into the bladder, are described in *Clinical relevance 3.3*.

CLINICAL RELEVANCE 3.3 ✚

The ureters normally run obliquely through the muscular wall of the bladder. This inferomedial course serves as a preventative mechanism against **vesico-ureteric reflux**. A congenitally defective 'flap valve' is responsible for primary vesico-ureteric reflux, typically diagnosed in infancy or childhood due to recurrent urinary tract infections (see *Clinical relevance 3.5*). Vesico-ureteric reflux may be considered a 'warning sign' for anomalies of the urinary tract, manifesting as chronic renal and systemic complications in later years due to parenchymal damage and renal impairment.

In relation to other structures, the ureters run anterior to the bifurcation of the common iliac arteries and then anterior to the internal iliac arteries (Fig. 3.2). In men, each ureter is posterolateral in relation to the corresponding vas deferens. In women, each ureter runs posterior to the corresponding ovary and inferior to the broad ligament (with the uterine arteries running along the base of the ligament). The close proximity of the ureters to the uterine arteries means that the former can easily be damaged during an operation to remove the uterus (**hysterectomy**).

Vasculature

The length of the ureter necessitates a blood supply from several arterial branches along its length:

- The proximal portion is supplied by the renal arteries
- The middle portion (within the abdominal cavity) is supplied by branches of the aorta, as well as the ovarian arteries in women and the testicular arteries in men
- The distal portion (within the pelvis) is supplied by branches originating from the common and internal iliac arteries – the most consistent amongst these is a branch from the internal iliac arteries called the inferior vesical artery.

Extensive vascular anastomoses exist along the length of each ureter.

Innervation

The ureters are innervated by several autonomic plexuses that surround the arteries which supply them, including the inferior and superior hypogastric, renal and aortic (testicular or ovarian) plexuses. The sympathetic fibres originate from the T10–L1 segments of the spinal cord, while the parasympathetic fibres are derived from the S2–S4 segments.

The function of the motor innervation is unclear. While it is not necessary for the normal peristaltic activity of the ureteric wall, it may serve to modify the activity of the smooth muscle cells. The sensory (afferent) fibres carry information pertaining to the level of distension of the ureters.

Lymphatic drainage

As with the vascular supply, there are several lymph drainage points along each ureter. The proximal ureter generally has vessels that drain into the lateral aortic nodes. Collecting vessels from the distal abdominal portion of the ureter usually carry lymph to the common iliac nodes. Lymph vessels from the pelvic part of the ureter will eventually drain into the common, external or internal iliac lymph nodes.

CLINICAL RELEVANCE 3.4 ✚

Common sites at which **ureteric calculi (stones)** may become lodged include the three points at which the ureters are anatomically narrowed along their course:

- Pelvi-ureteric region
- Pelvic brim (skeletal pelvis)
- Point of entry into the bladder.

Aetiology –

Calculus formation in the lower urinary tract can be due to:

- ↑ Solute concentration of urine
- pH disturbances
- ↓ Fluid passing through (particularly affecting individuals who do not drink adequate amounts of fluid).

Urinary tract stone formation has a preponderance for males (M:F ≈ 2:1). Other predisposing factors include:

- Urinary tract infections
- Primary metabolic disorders
- Urinary stasis.

Clinical presentation and complications –

Although often asymptomatic, clinical features include:

- Pain
- Haematuria
- Urinary tract infection (acute loin tenderness, pyrexia and septicaemia)
- Urinary tract obstruction.

A stone can impact in the wall of the ureter, obstruct urinary flow and induce an inflammatory response. This typically presents as loin or flank pain which can vary in nature (see *Points of interest 3.1*). The pain may radiate to the top of the thigh in women, and to the scrotum and penis in men (Fig. 3.8). Stasis of urine can result from outflow obstruction, creating an ideal environment for bacteria to grow and ascend along the ureter to eventually infect the kidney, termed pyelonephritis (see Ch. 5).

Acute obstruction of the ureter causes pain which typically radiates from the flank to the groin and iliac fossa (termed 'loin-to-groin' pain). The pink regions in Figure 3.8 indicate the general sites of referred pain from the kidneys and ureters. Distension of the renal pelvis and ureter can cause severe renal pain known as renal colic. Renal colic is not a true colicky pain because it is constant and unremitting.

REMEMBER !

Pain arising from an organ (viscus), radiates to the dermatome level which receives sensory nerve fibres from that organ. This is known as 'visceral referred pain'. Renal pain and ureteric pain are referred to:

- Small of the back (posterior to sacrum, above natal cleft)
- Flank/Loin (corresponds to lumbar region of the abdomen)
- Groin (inguinal region)
- Genitals.

POINTS OF INTEREST 3.1

Pain is characterised by specific features that should be ascertained from the patient's medical history:

Site
Onset (e.g. sudden or gradual)
Character (e.g. dull, sharp, 'stabbing')
Radiation
Associated features
Timing (e.g. constant or intermittent)
Exacerbating (and relieving) factors
Severity

This framework for taking a 'pain history' is often remembered by the mnemonic 'SOCRATES'. Signs and symptoms reported by patients provide clinicians with important clues for making diagnoses.

CLINICAL RELEVANCE 3.5 ✚

Lower urinary tract infections (UTIs) are usually caused by *Escherichia coli* (*E. coli*), *Proteus species* (*P. spp*) or other Gram negative coliform bacteria. Women are more susceptible to UTIs than men, due to the short female urethra which permits bacterial ascent and invasion of the urinary tract. Children and men who are found to be susceptible to UTIs should undergo investigations to identify any underlying abnormality of the urinary tract. It is important to determine the cause of recurrent UTIs because they can cause renal scarring, which may lead to chronic renal failure (see *Clinical relevance 3.2*) and hypertension.

Typical symptoms of UTI include loin pain (back pain), fever, 'lower urinary tract symptoms' including pain on micturition (dysuria), increased frequency and urgency in passing urine. UTI spread into the kidney causes pyelonephritis (see Ch. 5).

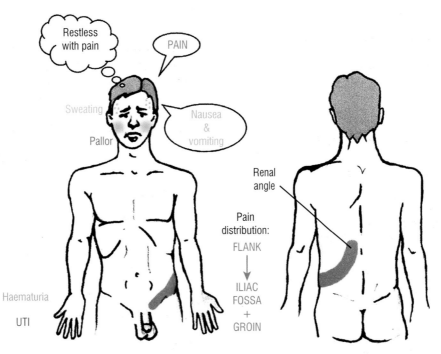

Figure 3.8 – Ureteric obstruction: Clinical presentation of the unwell patient

> **REMEMBER** !
>
> Infection of the lower urinary tract:
> - may be entirely asymptomatic
> - always carries the risk of spread to the kidneys.

KEY POINTS 3.2 🗝

Gross anatomy: Ureters

Each ureter is typically 25–30 cm long and 3 mm in diameter.

The ureters emerge from the renal pelvis and drain into the urinary bladder.

The ureters have muscular walls composed of smooth muscle cells, suited for peristalsis.

The ureters are mostly retroperitoneal.

Structural relations:

	Left ureter	Right ureter
Anteriorly	Sigmoid colon	Duodenum
	Sigmoid mesocolon	Terminal ileum
	Left colic vessels	Right colic and ileocolic vessels
	Left testicular or ovarian vessels	Right testicular or ovarian vessels
		Root of small intestine mesentery
Posteriorly	Psoas muscle (separates ureters from lumbar transverse processes)	
	Bifurcation of right common iliac artery	

Arterial supply to ureters –
- Upper part: Renal artery
- Middle part (in abdominal cavity): Testicular or ovarian artery
- Lower part (in pelvis): Superior vesical artery.

Venous drainage –
Veins correspond to the arteries (e.g. the renal veins drain the upper portion of the ureters).

Lymph drainage –
- Lateral aortic nodes
- Iliac nodes.

Nerve supply –
Autonomic plexuses:
- Renal
- Testicular or ovarian
- Hypogastric.

Sympathetic fibres (T10–L1)
Parasympathetic fibres (S2–S4)

The ureters can have stones lodged within them, resulting in stasis of urine which increases the risk of developing urinary tract infections.

Adrenal glands

The adrenal glands are a pair of yellow-brown retroperitoneal organs, one lying on the upper/superior pole of each kidney, hence the alternative name of 'suprarenal glands'. They are found in the posterior abdomen, typically at the level of the twelfth thoracic vertebra (T12), although the right adrenal gland is slightly lower due to the presence of the right lobe of the liver.

The right adrenal gland is 'pyramid-shaped' and smaller than the left. The left adrenal gland is crescentic in shape. There is some variability in the size and weight of these glands between individuals. The average adrenal gland measures 4–6 cm in length, 1–2 cm in width, and 3–4 cm in thickness. The adrenal glands have a combined mass of 8–10 g. The adrenal cortex makes up the vast majority (about 80%) of the volume of the gland (Fig. 3.14).

The adrenal glands are surrounded by fibrous renal fascia and a thick layer of peri-renal fat that serves a protective purpose and also separates the adrenals from the kidneys. Anterior to the right adrenal gland is the right lobe of the liver and inferior vena cava, and immediately posterior is the right crus of diaphragm. Anterior to the left adrenal gland is the lesser sac, stomach and pancreas, while posteriorly there is the left crus of diaphragm.

Blood supply

The adrenal glands have one of the highest rates of blood flow per gram of tissue. The adrenal (suprarenal) arteries supply the adrenals (Fig. 3.2). The superior, middle and inferior adrenal arteries originate from the inferior phrenic arteries, abdominal aorta and renal arteries, respectively.

One vein (the adrenal vein) exits the hilum of each adrenal gland and returns blood to the venous circulation. The right adrenal vein drains into the inferior vena cava while the left empties into the left renal vein (a similar anatomical organisation is found with the endpoints of the gonadal veins).

Nerve supply

There is a rich supply of pre-ganglionic sympathetic nerves to the adrenals, originating from the coeliac and renal nerve plexuses and terminating in the adrenal medulla. The secretion of adrenaline and noradrenaline (catecholamines) from the adrenal medulla occurs via sympathetic stimulation from the hypothalamus.

> **REMEMBER** !
>
> The adrenal medulla is a modified sympathetic ganglion. Its hormone output is predominantly adrenaline (about 85%) and noradrenaline, which are closely related chemically.

KEY POINTS 3.3

Gross anatomy: Adrenal glands

The adrenal glands sit above the kidneys. They are surrounded anteriorly by intra-abdominal structures and posteriorly by diaphragm.

The blood supply is from the adrenal arteries, listed below with their origins:

- Inferior phrenic arteries → Superior adrenal artery
- Abdominal aorta → Middle adrenal artery
- Renal arteries → Inferior adrenal artery.

Venous drainage of the adrenal glands:

- Right adrenal vein → IVC
- Left adrenal vein → Left renal vein.

The adrenal medulla is innervated by sympathetic nerve fibres.

The adrenal cortex is largely regulated by pituitary ACTH (see *Key points 3.9*).

SURFACE ANATOMY

There are not many palpable structures in the lower posterior abdominal wall, but normal bony landmarks can be useful for the clinician performing a physical examination. The surface anatomy of these structures is shown in Figure 3.9.

The kidneys are usually found just lateral to the spine in relation to ribs 11 and 12. Due to the presence of the large right lobe of the liver, the right kidney is slightly lower than the left:

- Left renal hilum – sits in the transpyloric plane, i.e. at the level of the first lumbar vertebra (L1), 5 cm lateral to the median plane
- Right renal hilum – usually below the transpyloric plane.

The proximal portion of each ureter begins at the hilum of the corresponding kidney, 5 cm lateral to the median plane at L1. From here they descend along approximately vertical lines.

Table 3.2 – Key anatomical features of the adrenal glands

	Left adrenal gland	Right adrenal gland
Location	Anterosuperior aspect of left kidney; approximately T12 vertebra level	Anterosuperior aspect of right kidney; slightly lower than left gland
Shape	Crescentic	Pyramidal
Arterial supply	Adrenal arteries	Adrenal arteries
Venous supply	Left adrenal vein → left renal vein	Right adrenal vein → inferior vena cava
Nervous supply	Coeliac and renal plexuses	Coeliac and renal plexuses
Anatomical relation to surrounding structures	Anterior: Lesser sac, stomach, pancreas Posterior: Left crus of diaphragm	Anterior: IVC (medial to gland) and liver (lateral to gland) Posterior: Right crus of diaphragm

The anatomical planes (median, sagittal, coronal and transverse) are shown on page 50.

The anatomical planes (median, sagittal, coronal and transverse) are shown on page 50.

CLINICAL RELEVANCE 3.6 +

Examination of the kidneys forms part of a complete abdominal examination. Techniques to confirm palpable kidneys include:

- Bimanual palpation and ballottement
  - by placing the palm of one hand over the lumbar region of the abdomen and the other hand posterior to the kidney at the back, pushing anteriorly
  - kidney mass descends in inspiration
- Percussion – often resonant note due to overlying colon (see *Key points 3.1*)
- Differentiate palpable spleen from left kidney

- Cannot feel deep to kidney mass
- Can insert fingers superficially (between kidney mass and costal margin)
- Kidney masses may be bilateral (e.g. polycystic kidneys are bilateral and irregular).

HISTOLOGY

Cellular morphology corresponds to the functional roles of different cell types. These cellular processes underlie homeostasis. Thus a basic knowledge of renal histology, alongside an understanding of gross anatomical features and their embryological origins, is important.

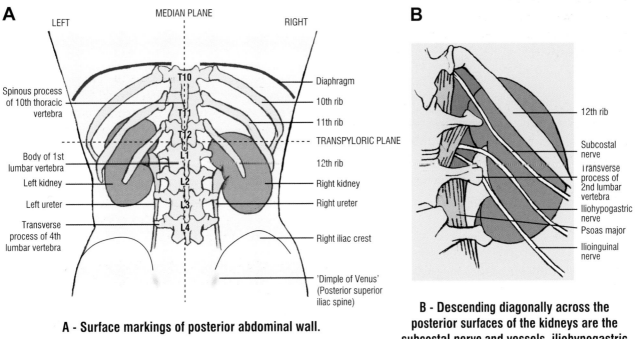

A - Surface markings of posterior abdominal wall.

B - Descending diagonally across the posterior surfaces of the kidneys are the subcostal nerve and vessels, iliohypogastric nerve and ilioinguinal nerve.

Figure 3.9 – Posterior view showing surface anatomy of kidneys and ureters

This section provides an overview of basic histological terms and concepts referred to in this chapter. Key cellular features and processes are defined.

Epithelial tissue (epithelium) is made up of cells characterised by:

- Cell polarity – distinct surface domains (apical, lateral and basal)

- Cell junctions – formed by specific cell-to-cell adhesion molecules

- Basement membrane – acellular, glycoprotein-rich layer underlying the basal cell surface.

These properties enable three principal functions of epithelium:

- Covering external body surfaces

- Lining internal body cavities

- Forming parts of glands.

The functional and morphological polarity of the three cell domains depends on:

- Specific biochemical cell surface features e.g. molecular composition of lipids and proteins

- Spatial arrangement of cells in the epithelium.

> **REMEMBER** !
>
> Classification:
>
> | | |
> |---|---|
> | **Simple** | One cell layer thick |
> | **Stratified** | Two or more cell layers |
> | **Pseudostratified** | Appears stratified but is actually a simple epithelium |
> | | |
> | **Squamous** | Cell width > height |
> | **Cuboidal** | Cell width ≈ height ≈ depth |
> | **Columnar** | Cell height > width |
> | **Transitional** | Specialised stratified epithelium that is able to distend |
>
> Key examples and typical locations:
>
> - Simple squamous epithelium – Bowman's capsule
>
> - Simple cuboidal epithelium – renal tubules
>
> - Columnar epithelium – zona glomerulosa (outer layer) of adrenal cortex
>
> - Transitional epithelium (urothelium) – lower urinary tract, from minor calyces of kidney to proximal portion of urethra.

The apical surface of renal tubule cells exhibits **microvilli** ('finger-like' cytoplasmic processes

extending from and increasing the area of the apical cell surface). The distinctive border of tightly packed vertical striations is termed 'brush border' due to its appearance in the light microscope. Cells may also have structural modifications known as **cilia** (motile cytoplasmic processes) emanating from and extending across the apical cell surface. Cilia appear as short, fine, 'hair-like' structures in the light microscope.

The lateral cell surface may display **plicae** (infoldings) which increase cell surface area, particularly at sites of fluid and electrolyte transport. The lateral cell surface is characterised by cell-to-cell adhesion molecules (unique proteins that constitute junctional specialisations). Three types of junctional complex are identified:

Occluding/Tight junctions (zonula occludens)

- Found on apical cell surfaces

- Impermeable, primary barrier to intercellular diffusion i.e. limiting movement of molecules between adjacent cells

- Tight junctions separate the luminal space from intercellular space, contributing to selective passage of substances across epithelium.

Anchoring junction (zonula adherens and macula adherens)

- Found on basolateral cell surfaces

- Provide structural/mechanical stability to epithelium (hence the name, 'anchoring')

- Two types: zonula adherens interacting with actin filaments, and macula adherens interacting with intermediate filaments.

Communicating/Gap junction

- Permit diffusion of small molecules between adjacent cells (e.g. ions, amino acids, sugars) enabling direct intercellular communication

- Allow co-ordination of cellular activity.

> **REMEMBER** !
>
> Movement of substances across epithelium occurs via two distinct pathways shown in Figure 3.10:
>
> **1** Paracellular pathway across tight junctions/zonula occludens between adjacent cells
>
> **2** Transcellular pathway across cell plasma membrane (mostly active transport).

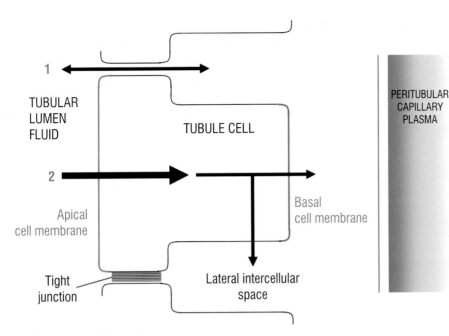

Figure 3.10 Paracellular and transcellular pathways for transport of substances across epithelium

The basal cell surface features:

Basement membrane

- Specialised structure underlying the connective tissue stroma that lies beneath the basal cell surface

- Composed of collagens, glycoproteins and proteoglycans which are extensively hydrated molecules with a high negative charge (the functional significance of these characteristics in glomerular filtration is described in Chapter 4).

Cell-to-extracellular matrix junctions

- Focal adhesions anchoring actin filaments into the basement membrane

- Hemidesmosomes anchoring intermediate filaments into the basement membrane.

Basal cell membrane infoldings

- ↑ Surface area of basal domain

- Particularly prominent at sites of fluid transport, e.g. proximal and distal renal tubules.

REMEMBER !

Each cell lining the tubule of the nephron has a 'luminal' membrane (apical surface) facing the tubular lumen, and a 'peritubular' membrane (basolateral surface) adjacent to the peritubular blood supply.

Cellular specialisations relate to specific cell functions.

Kidneys

Nephron

The nephron is the fundamental structural and functional unit of the kidney where urine formation occurs. Each human kidney contains approximately 1–2 million nephrons. These are hollow tubes composed of a single cell layer. Each nephron consists of a renal corpuscle and a tubular system comprising the proximal tubule, loop of Henle and distal tubule (Fig. 3.11). The collecting duct system is responsible for the final concentration of urine, and for simplicity will be considered the final part of the nephron. Up to eight nephrons may drain into a collecting duct.

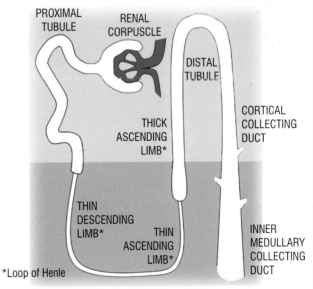

Figure 3.11 – General organisation of the nephron

Organisation of the nephron

This section provides an overview of the general organisation of the nephron. The actual organisation is more complex.

The renal corpuscle –

The renal corpuscle is the spherical structure at which the nephron begins. It comprises the glomerulus and Bowman's capsule. The glomerulus consists of a ball of 10–20 capillary loops surrounded by Bowman's capsule, which is a double-layered tubular epithelial invagination that forms the closed end of the tubular system. The renal corpuscle has a vascular pole where the afferent and efferent glomerular arterioles enter and exit Bowman's capsule respectively, and a urinary pole where the proximal convoluted tubule begins. The structure and function of the renal corpuscle is described in detail in Chapter 4.

Tubular system –

The tubular system of the nephron follows on from Bowman's capsule. Its segments are listed below and considered sequentially in Tables 3.4–3.8:

- Proximal convoluted tubule

- Loop of Henle
  (thick descending limb → thin descending limb → thin ascending limb → thick ascending limb)

- Distal convoluted tubule

- Collecting duct.

Brief notes on the histophysiology of each tubular segment are provided below. For detailed physiology of the renal tubular system see Chapter 5.

Types of nephron

There are different types of nephron, distinguished by the location of their renal corpuscles in the cortex.

There are cortical and juxtamedullary nephrons. Cortical nephrons make up the majority of the total nephron count, and can be further subdivided as shown in Table 3.3.

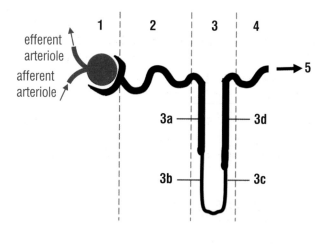

A.
1. Renal corpuscle: glomerulus + Bowman's capsule
2. Proximal convoluted tubule
3. Loop of Henle: (a) Thick descending limb/proximal straight tubule, (b) Thin descending limb, (c) Thin ascending limb, (d) Thick descending limb/distal straight tubule
4. Distal convoluted tubule
5. Collecting duct

Table 3.3 – Comparison of cortical and juxtamedullary nephrons

Type of nephron		Location of renal corpuscles	Relative length of structures
Cortical nephron	*Subcapsular*	Outer cortex	Short loops of Henle
	Intermediate	Mid-region of the cortex	Intermediate length of loops of Henle
Juxtamedullary nephron		Close to the base of a medullary pyramid	Long loops of Henle and long ascending thin segments

Table 3.4 – Histophysiology of the proximal convoluted tubule

Ultrastructure	Key features
Specialised cuboidal cells	
Brush border (microvilli)	A well developed glycocalyx (cell coat) containing ATPases, peptidases and disaccharides covers microvilli enabling reabsorption of amino acids, sugars and polypeptides
	Deep tubular invaginations between microvilli (covered with glycocalyx) are the site of protein endocytosis
Junctional complex	Zonula occludens and zonula adherens
Plicae (folds)	Lateral surface of cells
Interdigitating basal processes of neighbouring cells	Microfilament bundles found in the interdigitating processes are thought to be involved in fluid reabsorption, via regulation of transmembrane proteins
Basal striations	Highly concentrated elongated mitochondria in the basal processes
Transmembrane proteins	
Na^+/K^+-ATPase pumps	Responsible for reabsorption of Na^+, driving water reabsorption
AQP-1	Small hydrophobic transmembrane protein belonging to a family of aquaporin water channels (see *Clinical relevance 3.7*)

Proximal convoluted tubule

The proximal convoluted tubule receives ultrafiltrate from Bowman's space. The cuboidal cells of the proximal tubule possess surface specialisations which facilitate absorption and transport (Fig. 3.12). Transmembrane proteins are responsible for fluid reabsorption.

Reabsorption of bicarbonate and secretion of blood-derived organic acids and bases in the proximal convoluted tubule, regulate the pH of ultrafiltrate.

KEY POINTS 3.4

Histology: Proximal tubule

The proximal convoluted tubule is characterised by:

- **Specialised cuboidal cells** – glycocalyx, microvilli, junctional complex (tight junctions and anchoring junctions), plicae, interdigitating processes, basal processes and mitochondria

- **Transmembrane proteins** – Na^+/K^+-ATPase pumps and AQP-1 water channels.

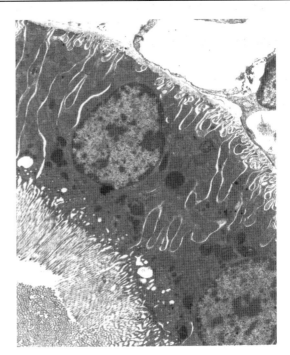

Figure 3.12 Electron micrograph of a group of cells of the proximal tubule

Visible at the cell apices are long microvilli and plicae (folds) are seen at the lateral surfaces. There are dense cytoplasmic lysosomes and mitochondria, and basal processes.
Image courtesy of Dr. Susan Anderson.

The reabsorption of every substance (including amino acids, glucose and water) is associated with active transport of Na^+, which relies on various cellular mechanisms ultimately dependent on the operation of Na^+/K^+-ATPase (see Ch. 5).

CLINICAL RELEVANCE 3.7 +

Research into aquaporin (AQP) water channel proteins may lead to the future development of therapeutic water channel blocking agents that could be of benefit in disorders of body fluid volume e.g. hypertension, congestive heart failure and cerebral oedema.

Loop of Henle

The loop of Henle is the site of reabsorption of approximately 25% of filtered NaCl and 15% of filtered water from the tubular lumen to plasma. The physiological role of the loop of Henle is described in Chapter 5. Key histological features are outlined in Table 3.5.

Loop of Henle	Relative permeability of tubular segment	
	Water	Solute
Thin descending limb	High	Low
Thin ascending limb	Low	High

Upon entering the thin descending limb, ultrafiltrate is isosmotic (relative to plasma). On leaving the thin ascending limb, the ultrafiltrate is hyposmotic. This makes sense given the different water and solute permeabilities of the two limbs, and the hypertonic extra-tubular environment (see Ch. 5). Osmolal concentration and tonicity are explained in Chapter 1.

KEY POINTS 3.5 ✍

Histophysiology: Loop of Henle

Thick descending limb
Cells are similar to those in the proximal tubule (specialised for absorption) but with a less complex morphology.

Thin descending and thin ascending limbs
Four types of epithelial cells are identified with morphological differences that probably reflect their different roles in the counter-current exchange mechanism of urine concentration (see Ch. 5):

- The thin descending limb is highly permeable to water. As ultrafiltrate passes through the thin descending limb it 'loses' water to the hyperosmotic interstitial fluid in the medulla.

- The thin ascending limb is highly permeable to solutes. As ultrafiltrate passes through the thin ascending limb it 'loses' ionic solutes to the interstitium.

- Ultrafiltrate leaves the loop of Henle to enter the distal convoluted tubule as a hyposmotic solution (relative to plasma).

Thick ascending limb
Large cuboidal cells specialised for solute reabsorption.

Distal tubule

The distal tubule is a relatively short segment of nephron (about a third of the length of the proximal convoluted tubule). The initial segment (early distal convoluted tubule) is considered separately to the late distal tubule.

The distal tubule and collecting duct system reabsorb just under 10% of filtered NaCl and a variable percent of water, as well as secreting K^+ and H^+.

Table 3.6 – Histophysiology of the distal tubule

Ultrastructure	Key features
Early distal convoluted tubule	Impermeable to water
	Reabsorption of Na^+ and secretion of K^+ (mediated by aldosterone)
	Reabsorption of HCO_3^- ions
	Secretion of ammonium (see Ch. 2)
Late distal tubule (initial collecting tubule)	Simple epithelium

Collecting tubules and collecting ducts

The distal tubules of two or more nephrons join in the cortex, forming a cortical collecting duct. This enters the medulla as the outer medullary collecting duct and travels further as the inner medullary collecting duct.

The collecting duct system is composed of two distinct types of cells – principal cells and intercalated cells. This includes the late distal tubule, i.e. the initial collecting tubule. The key histological features are described in Table 3.8. The physiological role of the collecting duct system is outlined in Chapter 5.

Table 3.5 – Histophysiology of the loop of Henle

Ultrastructure	Key features
Thick descending limb	Cells are not as specialised for absorption as those of the proximal convoluted tubule, with similar but fewer and less complex specialisations
Thin segment	Type I–IV epithelial cells are shown in Figure 3.13
Thin descending limb	High permeability to water
	Lower permeability to solutes
	Diffusion (passive movement) of water out of nephron into hyperosmotic interstitial fluid
Thin ascending limb	Impermeable to water
	High permeability to NaCl, permitting its passive diffusion into the interstitium
	Cl^- diffuses into the interstitium down its concentration gradient through Cl^--conducting channels
	Electrochemical neutrality is maintained by passive movement of counter ions (Na^+ and K^+) into the interstitium
	These transport processes are responsible for the hyperosmolarity of the interstitium, which directly relates to the movement of water out of the preceding nephron segment (see above – Thin descending limb)
Thick ascending limb	Ion transport from tubular lumen to interstitium
Large cuboidal cells	Apical nuclei
	Extensive basolateral plications (infoldings)
	Mitochondria associated with basal folds
	Fewer and less well developed microvilli compared with thick descending limb
Luminal (apical) cell membrane	$1Na^+/1K^+/2Cl^-$ symporters permit cellular entry of these ions from the lumen
	K^+ channels allow leakage of some K^+ ions back into the tubular lumen
	Positive gradient drives reabsorption of many other ions such as Mg^{2+} and Ca^{2+} via paracellular diffusion (Fig.3.10)
Basolateral cell membrane	Na^+/K^+-ATPase pumps (active transport of Na^+ out of the cell)
	Cl^- and K^+ channels allow these ions to diffuse out of cells

Table 3.7 – Histology of the collecting tubules and collecting ducts

Ultrastructure	Key features
Collecting tubules	Simple epithelium
Collecting duct system	Simple epithelium
Cortical collecting ducts	Cells with a flattened morphology (squamous to cuboidal)
Medullary collecting ducts	Cuboidal cells
	Transition to columnar cells with increasing duct size

KEY POINTS 3.6

Histology: Distal tubule and Collecting ducts

The distal tubule is considered in two parts:

- **Early distal tubule –**
  - Na^+ reabsorption and K^+ secretion (aldosterone-mediated)
  - HCO_3^- reabsorption
  - Ammonium secretion

- **Late distal tubule –**
  - Simple epithelium
  - Forms the initial collecting tubule (see below).

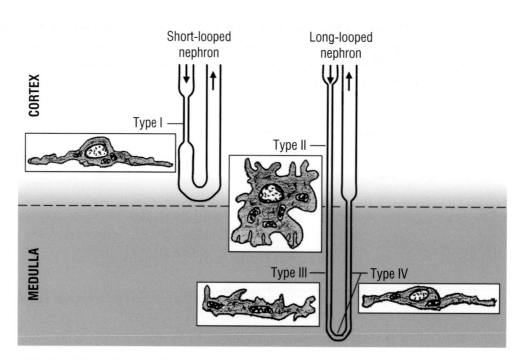

Figure 3.13 – Schematic diagram of epithelial cells in the thin segment of the loop of Henle

The diagram simply shows the location and morphology of individual epithelial cells. However epithelial cells *in situ* have neighbouring cells with which they form the epithelium, and their basal surface is attached to an underlying basement membrane.

Multiple nephrons drain into a collecting duct. The late distal tubule and collecting duct are characterised by:

- Simple epithelium

- **Principal (P) cells** –
  - Pale-staining
  - Surface specialisations including basal infoldings
  - Small mitochondria
  - Water permeability (ADH-regulated channels, AQPs)

- **Intercalated (IC) cells** –
  - Dark-staining
  - Abundant mitochondria
  - Surface specialisations including microvilli and basal interdigitations
  - Involved in acid-base balance (see Ch. 2).

Renal capsule

The renal capsule is a fibrous capsule of connective tissue that surrounds the kidney close to its surface. It is one of four coverings that support the organ. The other three layers are peri-renal adipose tissue, renal fascia and para-renal adipose tissue. The renal capsule is made up of an outer layer and an inner layer. The distinct histology of the two layers is considered in Table 3.9.

Loop of Henle epithelium	Location	Morphology
Type I	*Short-looped nephrons:* Thin descending limb Thin ascending limb	Thin, simple epithelium
Type II	*Long-looped nephrons:*	Specialised cells:
	Thin descending limb	Abundant cellular organelles (e.g. numerous small microvilli)
		Variable lateral interdigitation
Type III	*Inner medulla:* Thin descending limb	Similar to Type II epithelial cells but less specialised
Type IV	*Long-looped nephrons:* At the curve of the loop Thin ascending limb	Low, flattened epithelium Cellular organelles are scarce

Table 3.8 – Histophysiology of principal cells and intercalated cells of the late distal tubule and collecting duct

Cell type	Key features
Principal cells	Light (pale-staining) cells
	True basal infoldings
	Monocilium (each cell possesses only one cilium)
	Relatively few short microvilli
	Small spherical mitochondria
	ADH-regulated water channels, responsible for water permeability of collecting ducts
	AQP-3 and AQP-4, specific aquaporins located in the basolateral cell membrane (see *Clinical relevance 3.7*)
Intercalated cells	Dark cells
	Dense appearance of cytoplasm with numerous mitochondria
	Micropliae and microvilli on luminal (apical) surface
	Basal interdigitations with adjacent cells
	Many vesicles in apical cytoplasm
α-*intercalated cells*	Active secretion of H^+ into the collecting duct lumen via ATP-dependent pumps present in the basolateral membrane
β-*intercalated cells*	Secretion of HCO_3^- into collecting duct lumen via Cl^-/HCO_3^- exchangers in the basolateral cell membrane

Table 3.9 – Histology of the renal capsule

Ultrastructure	Key features
Outer layer	Dense connective tissue
	Fibroblasts (relatively few, with narrow elongated nuclei)
	Collagen fibres
Inner layer	Myofibroblasts (large numbers with round or elongated nuclei) The contractility of this cellular component is thought to oppose changes in volume and pressure occurring within the kidney
	Collagen fibres (relatively sparse)

REMEMBER

	Cortex	Medulla
Renal corpuscles	✓	✗
Convoluted tubules	✓	✗
Thick limbs of loop of Henle	✓	✓
Collecting tubules	✓	✗
Collecting ducts	✓	✓
Vascular supply	✓ (extensive)	✓

Renal cortex and medulla

Each kidney has a dark brown outer cortex and a light brown inner medulla (see *Points of interest 3.3*). Both regions contain the following structures – thick descending and thick ascending limbs of the loop of Henle, collecting ducts, blood vessels, lymphatics and nerves. Only the cortex contains renal corpuscles, convoluted tubules of nephrons and the collecting tubules. These differences between the two regions are summarised below.

POINTS OF INTEREST 3.3

At rest, about 25% of cardiac output supplies the two kidneys. The majority of blood flowing through the kidney is in the cortex (approximately 90–95%), with the remainder in the medulla. The difference in the distribution of blood within this organ is reflected in the colour seen in these two regions in the hemisected kidney.

Lobes and lobules

A **lobe** of the kidney consists of a single medullary pyramid and the portion of surrounding cortical material immediately adjacent to the sides and base of the pyramid (Figs. 3.2 and 3.4). There are 8–18 lobes in a human kidney (and an equal number of medullary pyramids).

Lobules are subdivisions of kidney lobes. A lobule is made up of:

- A central medullary ray (which contains a collecting duct and the group of nephrons draining into it)

- The cortical tissue associated with the medullary ray.

Interstitium

Renal connective tissue (interstitial tissue) surrounds nephrons and vessels (blood and lymphatic), accounting for over 20% of the renal medulla, but only ~5% of the renal cortex.

Endocrine components

Erythropoietin –
The major stimulus for the production of red blood cells (erythrocytes) is the glycoprotein erythropoietin, produced primarily by fibroblast-like cells in the renal interstitium.

Renin –
Regulation of blood pressure and maintenance of a euvolaemic state by the Renin-Angiotensin-Aldosterone system (see Ch. 1) relies on the acid protease enzyme renin, synthesised and secreted by granular cells. These are modified smooth muscle cells of the afferent arteriole, found in the juxtaglomerular region of the renal corpuscle (see Ch. 4). Granular cells contain spherical nuclei and secretory granules, compared with typical smooth muscle cells which possess elongate nuclei.

Vitamin D –
Vitamin D is activated by successive hydroxylation reactions, first in the liver and then the kidneys. The proximal tubule enzyme 1α-hydroxylase catalyses the conversion of the steroid precursor produced in the liver to its bioactive form 1,25-dihydroxycholecalciferol. This conversion is primarily regulated by parathyroid hormone, which activates 1α-hydroxylase. An overview of phosphate and calcium homeostasis is provided in Chapter 5.

REMEMBER !

- Erythropoietin is produced in the renal interstitium and stimulates red blood cell production

- Renin is released by the juxtaglomerular apparatus

- Vitamin D is activated by successive hydroxylations in the liver and kidneys.

KEY POINTS 3.7

Histology: Summary

The nephron is the structural and functional unit of the kidney, responsible for urine production.

Two types of nephrons are identified, based on the location of their renal corpuscles in the cortex – cortical nephrons and juxtamedullary nephrons.

The afferent glomerular arteriole supplies the glomerulus and the efferent glomerular arteriole drains the glomerulus (see Ch. 4).

The peritubular capillary network:

- Arises from the efferent arteriole

- Supplies the tubule of the nephron.

The predominant cell-type in the proximal convoluted tubule is cuboidal, with specialisations associated with absorption and fluid transport.

The proximal convoluted tubule is the initial and major site of reabsorption of filtered water and solutes.

The loop of Henle is responsible for the conversion of ultrafiltrate from an isosmotic to a hyposmotic solution.

The concentration of urine is modified along the distal convoluted tubule by variable reabsorption of water and solutes.

Exchange of Na^+ for K^+ in the distal convoluted tubule is regulated by aldosterone.

The collecting ducts are responsible for final urine concentration.

The renal cortex and medulla contain:

- Thick descending and thick ascending limbs of the loop of Henle

- Collecting ducts

- Blood vessels
- Lymphatics and nerves.

Only the cortex contains:

- Renal corpuscles
- Convoluted tubules (proximal and distal)
- Collecting tubules.

Ureters

The ureters are muscular tubes that allow drainage of urine from the kidneys to the bladder. The lumen of each ureter is typically 'star-shaped' and lined with transitional epithelium (urothelium). The urothelium is stratified (normally 3–5 cells thick) with the cells closest to the lumen having a cuboidal (or even rounded) appearance normally, but transforming into a squamous form when under compression i.e. when the ureters are distended by urine. This layer is impermeable to the urine passing through it (see *Points of interest 3.4*).

The lamina propria is a layer of dense collagen fibres that underlies the urothelium. It is elastic in nature, adding to the compliance of the ureters. The lamina propria and urothelium together form the **mucosal** layer of the ureters.

The next layer beyond the mucosa is the **muscularis**, which is made up of layers of smooth muscle cells. Contraction of the muscularis gives the lumen its usual 'star-like' appearance. Along the proximal two-thirds of the ureter, the muscularis consists of an inner longitudinal layer and an outer circular layer. However in the distal third, the muscularis exists as a three-layered structure with inner longitudinal, middle circular and outer longitudinal layers.

The outermost layer of the ureters is the **adventitia**. It is composed of connective tissue which surrounds the ureters and allows adherence to neighbouring structures.

Adrenal glands

The adrenal glands are a pair of yellowish retroperitoneal organs, one lying on the upper pole of each kidney on the posterior abdominal wall, typically at the level of T12. Each adrenal gland may be divided into cortex and medulla based on embryonic origin, functional characteristics and histological appearance (Fig. 3.14). The properties of the two regions are so distinctive that each adrenal gland is essentially two glands in one!

Adrenal cortex

The adrenal cortex can be subdivided into three regions based on histological appearance and function:
- Zona glomerulosa (outer layer)
- Zona fasciculata (middle layer)
- Zona reticularis (inner layer).

The different regions of the cortex secrete glucocorticoids, mineralocorticoids, and androgens (sex hormones, also known as gonadocorticoids). Hormonal secretion is under neuroendocrine control by the:

- Pituitary gland e.g. release of adrenocorticotrophic hormone (ACTH)
- Hypothalamus
- Renin-Angiotensin-Aldosterone system.

These regulatory mechanisms are summarised in Table 3.10. It should be noted that non-hormonal control mechanisms also exist, e.g. plasma $[K^+]$ influences aldosterone secretion.

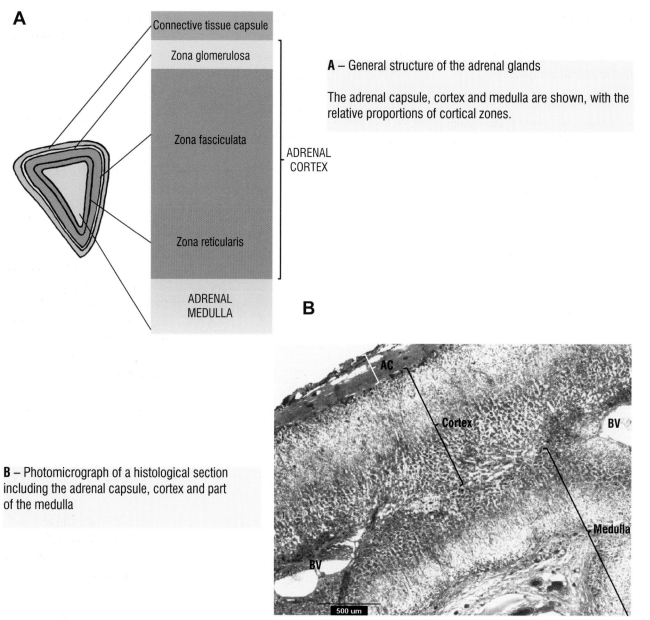

A – General structure of the adrenal glands

The adrenal capsule, cortex and medulla are shown, with the relative proportions of cortical zones.

B – Photomicrograph of a histological section including the adrenal capsule, cortex and part of the medulla

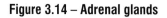

AC = Adrenal capsule   BV = Blood vessels

Figure 3.14 – Adrenal glands

Table 3.10 – Summary of neuroendocrine regulation of adrenal hormonal output

Controller mechanism	Adrenal cortex region	Response
Pituitary ACTH release (stimulated by hypothalamic corticotrophin-releasing hormone)	Zona fasciculata	↑ Glucocorticoid secretion Long-term: growth of zona fasciculata
	Zona reticularis	↑ Androgen secretion Long-term: growth of zona reticularis
Increased activity of Renin-Angiotensin-Aldosterone system	Zona glomerulosa	↑ Mineralocorticoid secretion Long-term: growth of zona glomerulosa

Zona glomerulosa –

- Thin layer immediately deep to the adrenal capsule, forming the outermost zone

- Makes up 10–15% of the volume of the adrenal cortex

- Consists of columnar cells arranged in oval clusters and irregular-shaped cords, surrounded by a rich supply of fenestrated capillaries

- Mineralocorticoids such as aldosterone are secreted here, and the cell ultrastructure correspondingly consists of copious levels of smooth endoplasmic reticulum (lipid droplets are sparse though)

- Aldosterone functions in the regulation of blood pressure, favouring sodium and water retention in the distal tubule of the nephron in the kidneys and other body sites, as well as decreasing reabsorption of potassium in the distal tubule (see Ch. 1).

Zona fasciculata –

- Middle zone of the cortex and thickest of all three sections

- Constitutes 75–80% of the volume of the cortex

- Cells in this layer are large and polyhedral, arranged in straight cords and separated by sinusoidal capillaries, and they have even more extensive smooth endoplasmic reticulum than the zona glomerulosa cells

- On histological slides zona fasciculata cells appear to have many vacuoles in the cytoplasm because they contain lipid droplets

- The cords are 1–2 cell(s) thick and project towards the direction of the adrenal medulla

- Glucocorticoids such as cortisol are secreted here, and have various important functions e.g. in stressful situations requiring increased glycaemic levels, glucocorticoids oppose insulin.

Zona reticularis –

- Innermost layer of the adrenal cortex

- Smallest of the three zones in terms of volume, making up just 5–10% of the cortex

- Cells in this layer are relatively small with more deeply staining nuclei and smooth endoplasmic reticulum but few lipid droplets

- The cells are arranged in cords with no uniform direction

- Anastomoses connect the cords which are separated by fenestrated capillaries running between them

- Cells of the zona reticularis principally secrete weak androgens (but also smaller amounts of glucocorticoids).

Adrenal medulla

The medulla forms the centre of the adrenal gland, and consists of:

- Parenchyma of epithelioid cells (chromaffin cells)

- Connective tissue

- Sinusoidal blood capillaries

- Nerves.

The epithelioid cells of the adrenal medulla (also known as chromaffin cells) are large and polyhedral. They are arranged in oval clusters and anastomosing cords, with intervening fenestrated capillaries (originating from cortical vessels), nerves and ganglion cells.

Chromaffin cells contain secretory vesicles of:

- Catecholamines (e.g. adrenaline, noradrenaline, dopamine)

- ATP

- Supporting proteins like chromogranin.

Upon stimulation by the numerous myelinated, pre-synaptic sympathetic nerve fibres, chromaffin cells secrete catecholamines into the bloodstream via nearby fenestrated capillaries (see *Clinical relevance 3.8*).

The ganglion cells of the adrenal medulla have axons that reach the adrenal cortex and modulate the secretion of endocrine substances in that part of the adrenal gland. Hormones of the adrenal cortex (e.g. glucocorticoids) influence the morphology of chromaffin cells in the medulla.

CLINICAL RELEVANCE 3.8

Chromaffin cells were previously also known as 'phaeochromocytes'. The term **phaeochromocytoma** is used to describe a catecholamine-secreting tumour composed of chromaffin cells, usually arising from the adrenal medulla. These uncommon neoplasms can cause hypertension which may be associated with other signs and symptoms of sympathetic innervation (e.g. tachycardia, tachypnoea, sweating).

KEY POINTS 3.9

Histology: Adrenal glands

The adrenal cortex is embryologically, functionally and microscopically different from the adrenal medulla.

The adrenal cortex secretes steroid hormones whereas the adrenal medulla is essentially a sympathetic ganglion and secretes catecholamines.

The adrenal cortex is considered in terms of three zones with distinct functions, summarised in the table below:

- Zona glomerulosa (outermost) – stimulated by Renin-Angiotensin-Aldosterone system

- Zona fasciculata (middle) – stimulated by pituitary ACTH release

- Zona reticularis (innermost) – stimulated by pituitary ACTH release.

REMEMBER !

Mineralocorticoids and glucocorticoids act in concert to prepare the body for the 'fight-or-flight' response.

EMBRYOLOGY

Embryology considers how tissues and organ systems develop in the embryo, thus enabling an understanding of normal anatomical variants and the many congenital pathologies (i.e. inherited or acquired conditions present at birth).

Urinary system

The normal, healthy human adult is equipped with two fully functioning kidneys. In reaching this stage the embryo develops 3 sets of kidneys in turn, of which the last (metanephroi) will mature and persist in the adult:

1. Pronephros   (plural: pronephroi)
2. Mesonephros (plural: mesonephroi)
3. Metanephros   (plural: metanephroi).

Pronephroi –
- Form in the 4th week of development
- Found in the neck region and made up of only a few cells
- Consist of pronephric ducts, which communicate with the cloaca
- Degenerate later on in the 4th week
- The pronephric ducts persist and form part of the mesonephroi.

Mesonephroi –
- Develop late in the 4th gestational week
- Functional until the end of the first trimester (12 weeks), with glomeruli and mesonephric tubules which drain into ducts that connect to the cloaca
- Lie caudal to the pronephroi
- Although these kidneys degenerate, parts are utilised in the male:
  - Mesonephric tubules form the testicular efferent ductules

Adrenal gland region	Primary hormonal secretion	Major regulatory functions
Adrenal cortex	Steroid hormones (cholesterol derivatives)	
Zona glomerulosa (~15% of cortex)	Mineralocorticoids e.g. Aldosterone	Electrolyte homeostasis Body fluid balance
Zona fasciculata (~80% of cortex)	Glucocorticoids e.g. Cortisol	Glucose and fatty acid metabolism Resistance to stress Suppression of immune and inflammatory responses
Zona reticularis (~5% of cortex)	Androgens e.g. Dehydroepiandrosterone (DHEA)	Masculinising effect (only with high serum levels)
Adrenal medulla	Catecholamines (amino acid derivatives) e.g. Adrenaline, noradrenaline	Sympathomimetic effects Conversion of glycogen → glucose Bronchodilatation ↓ digestion and urine production

- Mesonephric ducts form parts of the epididymis as well as the vas deferens and seminal glands.

Metanephroi –

• Develop in the 5th gestational week

• Function from the 9th week onwards.

The metanephric kidneys are derived from 2 sources which contribute to the structure of the permanent set of kidneys seen in the adult:

• Metanephric diverticulum (ureteric bud)

• Metanephric mass of intermediate mesoderm (Fig. 3.15 - overleaf).

The metanephric diverticulum begins development near the junction of the mesonephric duct and cloaca. As it elongates in the cranial direction, the diverticulum gives rise to the ureter, renal pelvis and collecting system.

The diverticulum invaginates the metanephric mass of intermediate mesoderm and progresses to divide and form the major calyces. It further divides to form the minor calyces and eventually the collecting tubules. At this time, the metanephric mass of intermediate mesoderm differentiates and forms nephrons – each consisting of a glomerulus and its accompanying proximal convoluted tubule, loop of Henle and distal convoluted tubule (Fig. 3.16). Each kidney develops approximately 1,000,000 nephrons which will continue to functionally mature after birth.

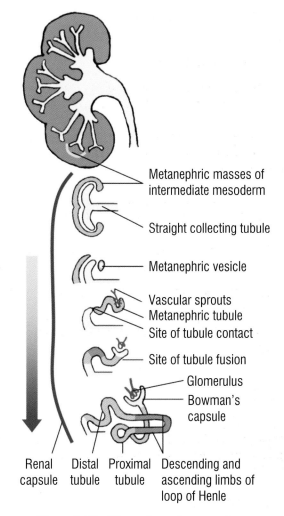

Figure 3.16 – Stages in nephrogenesis

Labels:
Metanephric masses of intermediate mesoderm
Straight collecting tubule
Metanephric vesicle
Vascular sprouts
Metanephric tubule
Site of tubule contact
Site of tubule fusion
Glomerulus
Bowman's capsule
Renal capsule
Distal tubule
Proximal tubule
Descending and ascending limbs of loop of Henle

CLINICAL RELEVANCE 3.9

Renal agenesis refers to the failure of kidney development in the fetus. Bilateral renal agenesis results in deficient formation of the amniotic fluid that surrounds and supports the fetus *in utero* (oligohydramnios). At birth, affected neonates are found to have **Potter's syndrome**, with abnormal facies and hypoplastic lungs. Bilateral renal agenesis occurs in 1 in 3000 births and is almost invariably fatal.

Positional changes of the kidney

In the developing fetus the kidneys change their position within the growing body (Fig. 3.17). The metanephric kidneys first develop in the pelvis and only reach their adult position by the 9th gestational week. This 'movement' along increasingly high cranial levels occurs because of relatively greater growth of the embryo caudal to the kidneys. Once at the right level, the kidneys rotate medially such that they attain their final adult anteromedial alignment.

Vasculature

As the kidneys ascend they require a change in blood supply to keep them nourished. Initially they rely on branches originating from the external iliac arteries. As they ascend, this then progresses to an arterial supply derived from the distal aorta, and subsequently aortic branches which are increasingly cranial in origin. The final branches come from the abdominal aorta at a point just inferior to the superior mesenteric artery (Fig. 3.2).

CLINICAL RELEVANCE 3.10

Horseshoe kidney is a condition in which the kidneys are fused in the midline, typically at the inferior poles (Fig. 3.18). The horseshoe kidney is limited in its embryological upward 'migration' by the root of the inferior mesenteric artery. The kidney may function as normal, but can be more susceptible to:

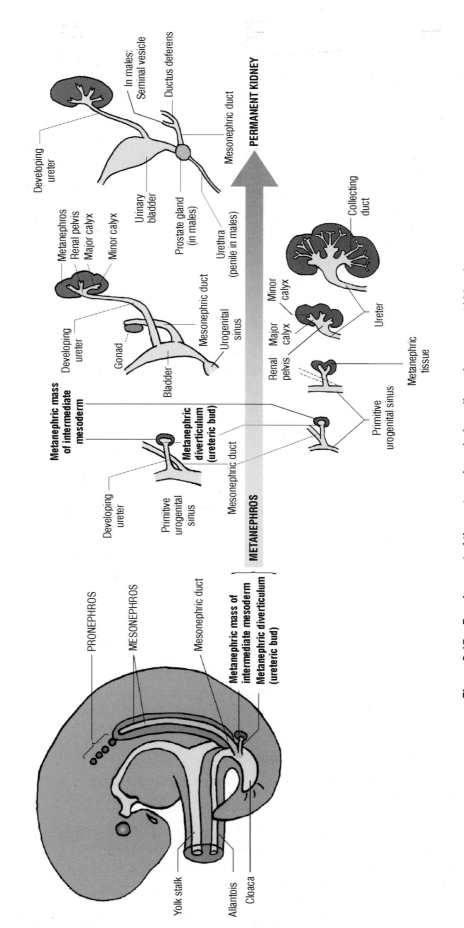

Figure 3.15 – Development of the metanephros (primordium of permanent kidney)

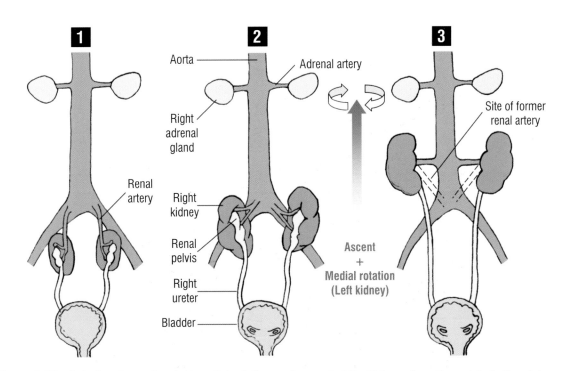

Figure 3.17 – Anterior views showing medial rotation and ascent of the kidneys from the pelvis to the abdomen

- Reflux (see *Clinical relevance 3.3*)

- Obstruction

- Recurrent infections (see *Clinical relevance 3.5*) – progressive renal scarring and obstruction can lead to hydronephrosis (back pressure resulting in dilatation of the renal pelvis and calyces)

- Calculus (stone) formation (see *Clinical relevance 3.4*).

Adrenal glands

The adrenal cortex is mesodermic in origin. It is first apparent at around 6 weeks of development as a collection of cells on each side, adjacent to the corresponding developing gonad. The cells of the fetal cortex come from the mesothelium which lines the posterior abdominal wall. These are soon encapsulated by a layer of mesenchymal cells from the mesothelium, which go on to form the permanent cortex. Differentiation of the cortical zones begins at the late fetal stage, with the zona reticularis not yet apparent at the time of birth.

The adrenal medulla is derived from the neural crest portion of the neuroectoderm (this is the same origin as that of post-ganglionic neurons of the sympathetic and parasympathetic nervous system). The adrenal medulla is first apparent at the 7th gestational week and is soon encapsulated by the fetal and early permanent cortices.

KEY POINTS 3.10

Embryology: Summary

Embryology: Kidneys and Ureters

Development of the kidneys begins in the 4th gestational week.

The first rudimentary kidneys are the pronephroi. These degrade towards the end of the 4th gestational week.

The mesonephroi are the intermediate set of kidneys which adopt the pronephric ducts as a part of their structure and function.

The final set of kidneys (metanephroi) progress to form the permanent set of kidneys. They are derived from the metanephric diverticulum and the metanephric mass of intermediate mesoderm.

Metanephric diverticulum → collecting system and ureters.

Metanephric mass of intermediate mesoderm → nephrons.

The metanephric kidneys originally develop in the pelvis and only reach their adult position by the 9th gestational week.

As the kidneys ascend, their blood supply changes:

- Branches of external iliac arteries (initial supply)

- Branches of aorta (distal → more cranial branches)

- Branches of abdominal aorta, just below superior mesenteric artery (final supply).

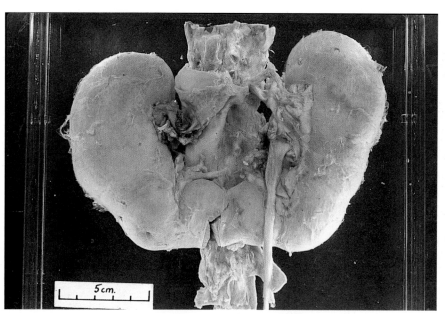

Figure 3.18 – Horseshoe kidney
Reprinted with permission from Alan Stevens, James Lowe and Ian Scott. Core pathology, 3ʳᵈ ed. Mosby, Copyright Elsevier (2008)

Renal agenesis is the failure of kidney development in the fetus.

Horseshoe kidney is when the kidneys are fused in the midline due to limited upward migration.

Embryology: Adrenal glands

Adrenal cortex:

• Derived from mesoderm

• First apparent ~ 6ᵗʰ gestational week

• Differentiation of cortical zones is a late process.

Adrenal medulla:

• Derived from neuroectoderm

• First apparent ~ 7ᵗʰ gestational week.

INTEGRATIVE CASE STUDY

A 35-year-old Caucasian male, PK, presents to his physician complaining of a sudden worsening of previous abdominal discomfort, with severe loin pain. He has also noticed that his urine appears bloody. He reports a family history of hypertension and his father had dialysis for end-stage renal failure.

On examination, PK is found to be hypertensive (BP = 180/100 mmHg) and the kidneys were enlarged and palpable bilaterally.

Blood test results: Serum creatinine = 282 mmol/L
[53 – 106 mmol/L]

Diagnosis?

• This is likely to be inherited **adult polycystic kidney disease**. In the case described above, cyst rupture is suspected, given the history of acute loin pain and haematuria.

• The pathogenesis, morphology and key clinical features of PKD are described in *Clinical relevance 3.1*.

• Diagnostic criteria vary with age and individual risk factors, but the presence of multiple cysts on ultrasonography is necessary (a single simple cyst is often a normal finding).

• As the condition is autosomal dominant with high penetrance, there is often a family history of PKD.

• There may be a family/personal history of brain aneurysm and stroke (due to ruptured intracranial aneurysm).

Further investigation?

In addition to serum creatinine, the following investigations should be considered:

- Full blood count (FBC).

- Urea and electrolytes.

- Urine microscopy and culture – adult PKD may present with urinary tract infection (*Clinical relevance 3.5*) including pyelonephritis (see Ch. 5).

- **Ultrasonography** (to establish diagnosis of PKD).

- Brain imaging for high risk groups.

Management?

- Anti-hypertensive medication (ACE inhibitors).

- Specific antibiotics to treat cyst infection.

- Patients should have:
  - Regular BP checks
  - Genetic counselling (if desired).

- The patient's children and siblings should be offered screening.

- Prognosis:
  - Autosomal dominant PKD is an important cause of chronic renal failure (*Clinical relevance 3.2*)
  - The main causes of death associated with adult PKD are renal failure and complications of hypertension.

Questions:

Gross anatomy: Kidneys

1. Are the following statements regarding the general structure of the kidney **true or false**?

   (a)   The renal substance can be divided into an inner cortex and an outer medulla.
   (b)   The renal papillae feed into major calyces, which fuse to form minor calyces and subsequently the renal pelvis.
   (c)   The kidneys are perfused by the renal arteries, with the right renal artery typically shorter than the left.
   (d)   The right renal vein is typically shorter than its left counterpart.
   (e)   The kidney is innervated by branches of the splenic plexus and the aortic plexus.

Gross anatomy: Ureters

2. Are the following statements regarding the general structure of the ureters **true or false**?

   (a)   Like the kidneys, the ureters are entirely retroperitoneal throughout their course.
   (b)   The ureters convey urine to the bladder via peristalsis of their thick muscular walls.
   (c)   Structures normally located anterior to the right ureter include sigmoid colon, colic vessels and gonadal vessels.
   (d)   The psoas muscle is normally situated posterior to the ureters, separating them from the transverse processes of thoracic vertebrae.
   (e)   The renal veins drain the upper portion of the ureters.

Gross anatomy: Adrenal glands

3. Are the following statements regarding the general structure of the adrenal glands **true or false**?

   (a)   Each adrenal gland sits on the upper pole of its respective kidney.
   (b)   The adrenal glands are innervated by sympathetic nerve fibres.
   (c)   The left adrenal gland typically lies posterior to the stomach.

Gross anatomy: Renal system vasculature

4. Match each structure to the appropriate statement, from the list below.

   i.   Abdominal aorta   iv.   Inferior vena cava
   ii.   Renal artery   v.   Left renal vein
   iii.   Right adrenal vein   vi.   Right renal vein

   (a) This structure supplies the middle adrenal artery.
   (b) This structure supplies the upper part of the ureters and the inferior adrenal artery.
   (c) The left adrenal vein drains into this structure, which also drains the upper part of the ureter.
   (d) The renal veins and the right adrenal vein drain into this structure.

Histology: Kidneys

5. Are the following statements regarding the nephron **true or false**?

(a) Two types of nephrons are identified, based on the location of their renal corpuscles in the cortex – cortical nephrons and juxtamedullary nephrons.
(b) Efferent glomerular arterioles drain the glomerular capillary network and eventually give rise to peritubular capillaries.
(c) The proximal tubule is characterised by simple columnar cells and transmembrane proteins.
(d) The thin ascending limb of the loop of Henle is highly permeable to water, permitting the movement of water out of the tubule lumen to enter the hyperosmotic interstitial fluid.
(e) Principal cells possess water channels, conferring water permeability to the collecting duct.

Histology: Ureters

6. Choose the most appropriate term from the list below, to complete the following statements.

i.	Urothelium	iv.	Hyaline cartilage
ii.	Collagen	v.	Muscularis
iii.	Connective tissue	vi.	Adipose tissue

(a) Each ureter is lined by three layers, of which the innermost is the mucosal layer, consisting of collagen and _____.
(b) The adventitia forms the outermost layer of the ureter wall and this contains _____.
(c) The _____ layer of the ureter wall is composed of circular and longitudinal layers of smooth muscle cells.

Histology: Adrenal glands

7. Match one structure from the list below, to the appropriate description.

i.	Zona glomerulosa	iv.	Adrenal medulla
ii.	Zona fasciculata	v.	Hypothalamus
iii.	Zona reticularis	vi.	Pituitary gland

(a) The outermost region of the adrenal cortex, responsible for mineralocorticoid secretion.
(b) Cortisol secretion from this structure is stimulated by adrenocorticotrophic hormone released by the pituitary gland.
(c) Hormones secreted by this structure directly cause increases in heart rate, sweating and airway dilatation.
(d) This structure accounts for a minority of the total volume of the adrenal cortex, primarily secreting androgen hormones.

Embryology: Renal system

8. Are the following statements regarding fetal development **true or false**?

(a) The kidneys normally begin their development as the pronephroi around the 4th gestational week.
(b) The mesonephroi are the final embryological set of kidneys that form the permanent kidneys, initially developing in the pelvis and reaching their adult position by the 9th gestational week.
(c) The collecting system and ureters are derived from the metanephric diverticulum.
(d) The external iliac artery is the only artery that directly supplies the developing kidney throughout its embryological ascent.
(e) 'Horseshoe kidney' refers to the failure of kidney development in the fetus.
(f) The adrenal cortex is derived from mesoderm.
(g) Differentiation of the cortical zones is an early process, with all three zones apparent at birth.

Answers:

(see *Key points 3.1*)

1. (a) False. The two distinct regions of the kidney are the outer cortex and the inner medulla.
   (b) False. Renal papillae → Minor calyces → Major calyces → Renal pelvis.
   (c) False. The right renal artery is typically longer than the left.
   (d) True.
   (e) False. The kidney is innervated by branches of the splanchnic plexus and the aortic plexus.

(see *Key points 3.2*)

2. (a) False. The ureters are mostly retroperitoneal.
   (b) True.
   (c) False. The sigmoid colon, colic vessels and gonadal vessels lie anterior to the left ureter.
   (d) False. The psoas muscle is found posterior to the ureters and separates them from the lumbar transverse processes.
   (e) True.

(see *Key points 3.3*)

3. (a) True.
   (b) True.
   (c) True.

(see *Key points 3.4 - 3.6*)

4. (a) i. Abdominal aorta.
   (b) ii. Renal artery.
   (c) v. Left renal vein.
   (d) iv. Inferior vena cava.

(see *Key points 3.7*)

5. (a) True.

  The juxtamedullary nephron is also characterised by a long loop of Henle with a long ascending thin segment. This is physiologically significant (see Ch. 5).

  (b) True.
  Filtrate reabsorbed from the tubular lumen re-enters the systemic circulation via peritubular capillaries.

  (c) False. The proximal tubule is characterised by specialised cuboidal cells and transmembrane proteins.
  This segment of the renal tubule forms the initial and major site of reabsorption of filtered water and solutes (see Ch. 5).

  (d) False. The thin ascending limb has a low water permeability.
  The statement is true of the thin descending limb, which is highly permeable to water.

  (e) True.

(see *Key points 3.8*)

6. (a) i. Urothelium (transitional epithelium).
   (b) iii. Connective tissue.
   (c) v. Muscularis.

(see *Key points 3.9*)

7. (a) i. Zona glomerulosa.

   (b) ii. Zona fasciculata.

   (c) iv. Adrenal medulla.
   Adrenaline secretion has sympathomimetic effects e.g. tachycardia and bronchodilatation.

   (d) iii. Zona reticularis.

(see *Key points 3.10* and *Clinical relevance 3.10*)

8. (a) True.

   (b) False. The mesonephroi are the intermediate set of kidneys, following the pronephroi.
   The metanephroi are the final set of kidneys that progress to form the permanent adult kidneys, originally developing in the pelvis and only reaching their adult position by the 9th gestational week.

   (c) True.
   (d) False. The blood supply to the kidneys changes during their upward migration. Branches of the external iliac artery provide the initial blood supply.

   (e) False. Horseshoe kidney is a condition in which the kidneys are fused in the midline due to abnormal upward migration (limited by the root of the inferior mesenteric artery).
   Renal agenesis is the failure of kidney development in the fetus.

   (f) True.
   The adrenal medulla is neuroectodermal in origin.

   (g) False. Differentiation of cortical zones is a late process. The zona reticularis is not apparent at birth.

CHAPTER 4 — RENAL CORPUSCLE

Written by: Sunita Deshmukh & Newton Wong

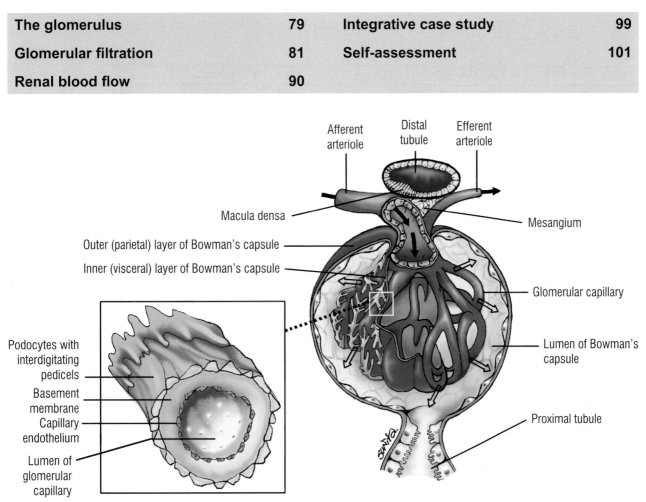

Figure 4.1 – Renal corpuscle
Black arrows indicate the direction of blood flow. Transparent arrows represent filtration.

The renal corpuscle includes the glomerulus and Bowman's capsule. The meeting of these two structures forms the site where constituents of the blood from the renal artery gain access to the tubular component of the nephron, forming the filtrate (Fig. 4.1).

THE GLOMERULUS

The glomerulus is the vascular component of the renal corpuscle. It is the site of initial filtration of blood arriving at the renal corpuscle, delivered by the afferent arteriole. The efferent arteriole carries the blood away following filtration at the glomerulus. The vascular supply is described in Chapter 3.

The glomerulus is formed by the collection of capillaries at Bowman's capsule. There is a pressure gradient at the site of filtration created by the difference in diameter of the afferent and efferent arterioles, the latter being slightly narrower and longer. The pressure head produces a driving force that tends to 'push' fluid into Bowman's space. Arteriolar diameter can be influenced by vasoactive substances, so the filtration pressure gradient and renal blood flow can be altered (Fig. 4.6).

Juxtaglomerular apparatus

The juxtaglomerular apparatus has two major components:

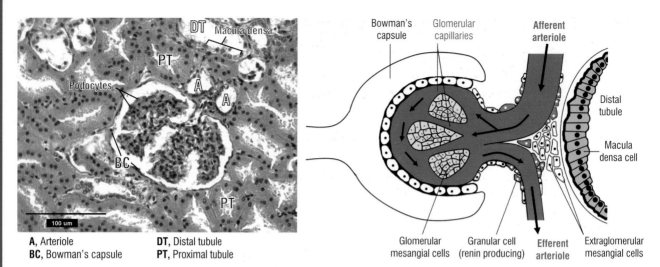

A, Arteriole **DT**, Distal tubule
BC, Bowman's capsule **PT**, Proximal tubule

A – Photomicrograph of an H&E-stained specimen showing a renal corpuscle

B – Schematic diagram showing the organisation of the juxtaglomerular apparatus

Figure 4.2 – Structure and organisation of the renal corpuscle

- Specialised vascular smooth muscle cells known as **granular cells**, found in the tunica media (middle layer of the wall) of afferent arterioles

- Specialised distal tubule cells forming the **macula densa** (Fig. 4.2). These cells detect changes in tubular fluid [NaCl].

The juxtaglomerular apparatus lies at the junction between the afferent and efferent arterioles, and the glomerulus (see *Points of interest 4.1*). On its route, the distal convoluted tubule approaches the hilar region of the renal corpuscle (where the afferent arteriole enters and the efferent arteriole leaves Bowman's capsule), enabling contact between the macula densa and a group of specialised mesangial cells. These cells and their matrix collectively occupy the interstitial space of the glomerulus, known as the **mesangium**.

Granular cells possess secretory granules containing the enzyme **renin**, which has important regulatory functions. The histology of granular cells is described in Chapter 3. Renin is released when there is:

- ↓ Na⁺ concentration in the tubular filtrate

- Sympathetic stimulation of granular cells.

Renin initiates the conversion of angiotensinogen to angiotensin I. The latter is then converted to angiotensin II by angiotensin converting enzyme (ACE). Angiotensin II stimulates:

- Vasoconstriction

- Na⁺ reabsorption in the renal tubule

- Aldosterone release from the adrenal glands.

Together with macula densa cells, granular cells play a role in the autoregulation of glomerular filtration rate (GFR).

The Renin-Angiotensin-Aldosterone System is described in Chapter 1.

Mesangium

Each glomerular capillary has a juxta-mesangial region effectively lacking a basement membrane (the basement membrane merges with the mesangial cell stroma). This creates an interface between mesangial cells and capillaries lined with vascular smooth muscle and fenestrated endothelium, permitting:

- passage of water, solutes and uncharged macromolecules from capillaries to mesangial cells

- a link between the macula densa (basolateral aspect of cells) and glomerular capillaries, via mesangial cells.

The role of glomerular mesangial cells in physiological and pathological conditions is not fully understood. Cell function appears to vary with cell location (Table 4.1). It is thought that glomerular mesangial cells probably contribute to the maintenance of the filtration membrane, and there is evidence for their involvement in the regulation of GFR.

Table 4.1 – Comparison of glomerular and extra-glomerular mesangial cells

	Mesangial cells	
	Glomerular	**Extra-glomerular**
Location	Situated between capillaries within the glomerulus	Lie outside the glomerulus between the afferent and efferent arterioles, adjacent to the macula densa
Function	Secrete prostaglandins that are important in the regulation of blood flow	Produce mesangial matrix
	Provide structural support, holding together the capillaries in each glomerular tuft	
	Phagocytosis	

POINTS OF INTEREST 4.1

'**Juxta**' is a prefix meaning 'near' or 'next to'. The term **juxta**glomerular apparatus describes the close proximity of this structure to the glomerulus.

KEY POINTS 4.1

The renal corpuscle is the initial part of the nephron.

The renal corpuscle consists of:

- Glomerulus

- Bowman's capsule.

A tuft of capillaries (surrounded by Bowman's capsule) forms the glomerulus, the initial site of filtration of the blood arriving at the nephron.

The afferent glomerular arteriole supplies the glomerulus and the efferent glomerular arteriole drains the glomerulus (see Ch. 3).

Afferent arterioles are shorter in length and wider in diameter compared to other arterioles, contributing to the glomerular pressure gradient that drives filtration.

The juxtaglomerular apparatus contains:

- Renin-secreting granular cells in the afferent arteriole wall – involved in the Renin-Angiotensin-Aldosterone system (see Ch. 1)

$$\text{Angiotensinogen} \xrightarrow{\text{Renin}} \text{Angiotensin I} \xrightarrow{\text{ACE}} \text{Angiotensin II}$$

- Macula densa cells in the distal tubule – detect changes in tubular fluid [NaCl] and act in concert with granular cells to maintain renal perfusion and blood pressure.

Mesangial cells are located in the glomerular interstitium and are involved in regulating glomerular filtration.

GLOMERULAR FILTRATION

Filtration pathway

Glomerular filtration occurs across three layers:

1. **Glomerular capillary wall**
2. **Basement membrane**
3. **Podocytes.**

The filtration pathway (Fig. 4.3) is summarised in Table 4.2.

1. Glomerular capillary wall

The vessel wall is a single cell-layer thick, formed by flattened endothelial cells. These cells are **fenestrated** with ultramicroscopic pores (~70 nm in diameter). The fenestrated nature of glomerular capillary endothelium means this membrane is significantly more permeable to water and solutes compared to other capillaries in the body. The maximum molecular weight of substances that can pass through is 70 kDa (see *Points of interest 4.2*).

2. Basement membrane

This **non-cellular** layer comprises:

- **Collagen**
- **Glycoproteins** (fibronectin and laminin).

The basement membrane is relatively thick and due to the presence of negatively-charged glycoproteins, this layer repels anionic proteins such as albumin. These negative charges (necessary for normal basement membrane function) may be disrupted in renal disease, permitting filtration of some lower molecular weight proteins. Examples of pathologies characterised by proteinuria (protein in the urine) are described in *Clinical relevance 4.1* and *4.9*.

3. Podocytes

These cells form the visceral (inner) epithelial layer of Bowman's capsule (Fig.4.1). Podocytes possess elongated processes that protrude from the basement membrane and the smallest of which are also called **foot processes** or pedicels. 'Podo' means 'foot', hence the name **podo**cyte is given to a cell with foot processes. Between the foot processes are **filtration slits** thought to confer size selectivity.

Therefore plasma constituents of suitable **molecular size** and **charge** pass through the filtration barrier easily (e.g. sodium and potassium ions, glucose, amino acids). However, plasma proteins, blood cells and thrombocytes (platelets) are not filtered.

POINTS OF INTEREST 4.2

'Fenestra' is the Latin word for 'window'. Endothelial fenestrae are porous openings found in specialised capillary endothelium of renal glomeruli, and also at some other tissue sites e.g. endocrine glands and intestinal villi.

KEY POINTS 4.2

Glomerular filtration takes place across 3 layers:

1. Glomerular capillary wall (fenestrae/pores)
2. Basement membrane
3. Podocytes of Bowman's capsule (filtration slits).

Glomerular filtration rate (GFR) measures how effective the filtration process is.

The passage of a molecule across the glomerular membrane (filtration barrier) is determined by its:

- Charge
- Size.

Substances that pass easily into Bowman's space are:

- Neutral or positively charged
- ≤ 8 nm in diameter.

Selective permeability of the barrier minimises passage of substances which are not normal constituents of the filtrate.

Anionic plasma proteins cannot normally pass through the filtration barrier because of specific properties of the basement membrane.

Net filtration pressure

The net pressure of glomerular filtration is driven by physical forces that determine the movement of fluid between plasma and interstitium, known as **Starling forces**:

1. Glomerular capillary hydrostatic pressure (P_G)
2. Plasma-colloid osmotic pressure (π_G)
3. Bowman's capsule hydrostatic pressure (P_B)
4. Bowman's capsule colloid osmotic pressure (π_B).

The influence of each of these forces on net filtration pressure is described below and summarised in Table 4.4. The Starling forces can be categorised:

- **Hydrostatic pressure** – exerted directly by water
- **Colloid-osmotic pressure** – due to protein concentration gradient across filtration membrane (see *Points of interest 4.3*).

Table 4.2 – Summary of the glomerular filtration pathway

	1	2	3
Layer	Glomerular capillary wall	Basement membrane	Visceral (inner) layer of Bowman's capsule
Route	Fenestral pores	Direct passage through this acellular layer	Filtration slits

Note that the journey of plasma constituents undergoing filtration is at no point intracellular.

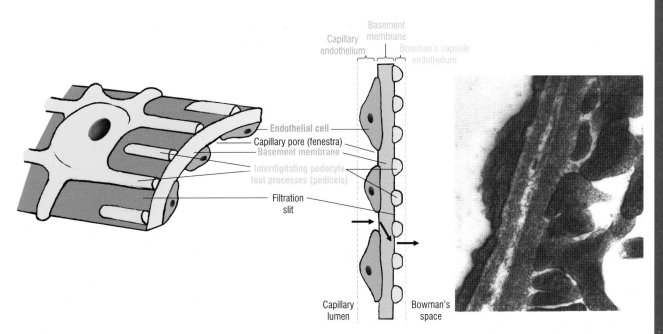

A – Diagram and electron micrograph showing the microscopic organisation of the glomerular (filtration) membrane

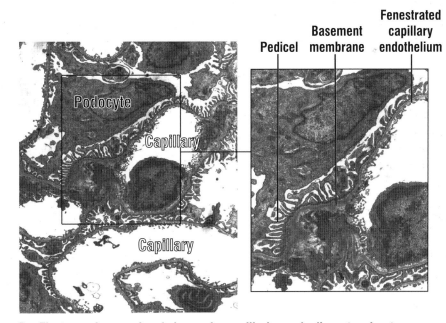

B – Electron micrographs of glomerular capillaries and adjacent podocytes

Figure 4.3 – Pathway of glomerular filtration

Three layers form the filtration barrier – capillary endothelium, basement membrane, and podocyte.
Electron micrographs courtesy of Dr. Susan Anderson.

Hydrostatic pressure is the pressure exerted by a fluid on a membrane (see Ch. 1). The magnitude of blood flow (Q) is influenced by:

- **Pressure (P)** i.e. force of flow across a given area
- **Resistance (R)** to flow (see equation 4.1).

$$Q = \frac{\Delta P}{R} \tag{4.1}$$

Q   = Blood flow

ΔP = Change in pressure across capillary beds (i.e. mean arterial pressure minus venous pressure for the organ)

R   = Resistance against blood flow through the organ

Fluid volume, viscosity and vessel length are also important considerations but under normal physiological conditions these remain relatively constant.

> **REMEMBER** !
>
> Starling forces determine fluid movement across the capillary wall, i.e. between the blood plasma and interstitial fluid. Body fluid compartments are described in Chapter 1.

POINTS OF INTEREST 4.3

Colloid osmotic pressure is commonly referred to as 'oncotic pressure'.

1. Glomerular capillary hydrostatic pressure

Glomerular capillary hydrostatic pressure is equivalent to the glomerular capillary blood pressure. Its determinants are identified in the table below.

Table 4.3 – Summary of factors that determine glomerular capillary hydrostatic pressure

Aspects of flow	Variable factors
Pressure (driving force)	**Cardiac output** The volume of blood ejected per unit time is controlled by stroke volume and heart rate
Resistance	**Afferent and efferent arterioles** (Fig. 4.6) The relatively narrow efferent arteriole creates a high resistance conveying two important properties to the pressure of glomerular capillary blood: - raised pressure - non-decremental pressure (see *Points of interest 4.4*)

> **REMEMBER** !
>
> Glomerular capillary hydrostatic pressure favours filtration and is the major driving force of glomerular filtration.

POINTS OF INTEREST 4.4

The non-decremental pressure of glomerular capillaries contrasts with other capillaries in the body, which display significant decreases in blood pressure along the length of the vessel.

2. Plasma-colloid osmotic pressure

In comparison to hydrostatic pressure (the pressure exerted by a fluid on a membrane), colloidal osmotic pressure arises due to the difference in solute concentration across the glomerular filtration membrane (specifically plasma proteins in the case of plasma-colloid osmotic pressure). This drives the osmotic movement of water down its concentration gradient (Fig. 4.4).

Figure 4.4 – Osmotic movement of water driven by plasma-colloid osmotic pressure

Water leaves **Bowman's capsule**
(region of higher water concentration due to absence of plasma proteins)
↓
Across the semi-permeable
glomerular membrane
↓
Enters the **glomerular capillaries** (region of lower water concentration due to presence of plasma proteins intravascularly)

This osmotic pressure opposes glomerular filtration pressure, and is estimated to be about 25–30 mmHg. Cellular transport processes (e.g. osmosis) are described in Chapter 1.

ASK YOURSELF 4.1 ?

Q. If there is excessive leakage of plasma proteins into the filtrate, as occurs in diabetic nephropathy (see *Clinical relevance 4.1*), what effect will this have on plasma-colloid osmotic pressure and thus on net filtration pressure?

A. Increased movement of plasma proteins from the blood into Bowman's capsule will reduce the difference in plasma protein concentration across the glomerular (filtration) membrane. This concentration gradient is usually responsible for maintaining plasma-colloid osmotic pressure. Since the plasma-colloid osmotic pressure opposes filtration, a significant decrease in its driving force will augment net filtration pressure.

3. Bowman's capsule hydrostatic pressure

The pressure of the fluid in Bowman's capsule (the initial part of the renal tubule) physically encourages movement of filtrate out of the capsule and thus opposes filtration.

Table 4.4 – Summary of the Starling forces and their effects on glomerular filtration

	Starling forces	Effect on filtration	Pressure
1	Glomerular capillary hydrostatic pressure (P_G)	**Promotes** filtration	~ 60 mmHg
2	Plasma-colloid osmotic pressure (π_G)	**Opposes** filtration	~ 25 mmHg
3	Bowman's capsule hydrostatic pressure (P_B)	**Opposes** filtration	~ 15 mmHg
4	Bowman's capsule colloid osmotic pressure (π_B)	Under normal conditions, π_B does not directly influence filtration pressure – it is practically zero, since glomerular ultrafiltrate is nearly protein-free	

Net filtration pressure is the resultant force based on this simple equation:

$$\begin{array}{ccccccc} \text{Net filtration pressure} & = & \text{Glomerular capillary hydrostatic pressure} & - & \text{Plasma-colloid osmotic pressure} & - & \text{Bowman's capsule hydrostatic pressure} \\ \\ 20\text{ mmHg} & = & 60 & - & 25 & - & 15 \end{array} \qquad (4.2)$$

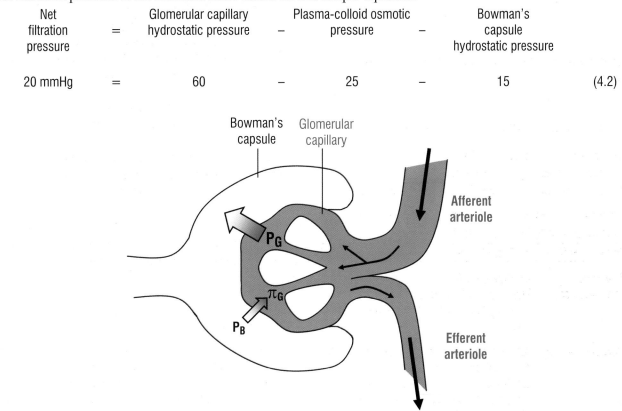

Figure 4.5 – Factors determining the net filtration pressure and their relative directions

CLINICAL RELEVANCE 4.1

People with type 1 and type 2 diabetes mellitus are susceptible to microvascular complications including glomerular pathology termed **diabetic nephropathy**, which manifests clinically as impaired renal function. The leading cause of renal failure is diabetes mellitus.

Following the onset of diabetes there may be excessive leakage of protein into the urine termed **microalbuminuria** (daily urinary excretion of 30–300 mg of albumin) which precedes overt **proteinuria**. Proteinuria is a measure of deteriorating renal function and is often a pre-indication of chronic renal failure which develops progressively (see Ch. 3).

The metabolic defect of insulin deficiency (resulting in glucose intolerance) and the microangiopathy occurring in diabetes mellitus, are closely associated with changes in renal morphology responsible for the pathogenesis of diabetic nephropathy:

- *Thickening of the glomerular capillary basement membrane*

  There are increases in collagen (type IV) and fibronectin. Typically there is also progressive mesangial widening and tubular basement membrane thickening.

- *Mesangial matrix expansion*

  Diffuse increase of mesangium is usually associated with glomerular capillary basement membrane thickening and worsening renal function.

- *Haemodynamic changes*

  Glomerular filtration rate (GFR) is typically raised in early diabetic nephropathy, with glomerular hypertrophy (increased glomerular filtration area and glomerular capillary pressure). However, GFR decreases in later stages of diabetes.

Prevention of systemic hypertension in patients with diabetes can have reno-protective effects. Two classes of drug found to be beneficial in the management of diabetic nephropathy are:

- **Angiotensin converting enzyme (ACE) inhibitors** (drug of choice for hypertensive diabetes patients) e.g. lisino**pril**, rami**pril**.

- **Angiotensin II receptor antagonists** e.g. lo**sartan**, val**sartan**. Angiotensin II acts on angiotensin AT1 receptors (there are two types of receptors i.e. AT1 and AT2).

Mechanisms of drug action with respect to the Renin-Angiotensin-Aldosterone System are described in *Clinical relevance 4.2*.

CLINICAL RELEVANCE 4.2 ✚

Angiotensin converting enzyme (ACE) inhibitors are an important class of drug for:

- Management of heart failure

- Anti-hypertensive medication.

ACE inhibitors lower blood pressure by inhibiting angiotensin converting enzyme, normally involved in the conversion of angiotensin I to angiotensin II (see Ch. 1). **Inhibition of angiotensin II** has the following effects:

- Vasodilatation (↓ total peripheral vascular resistance)

- ↓ Na⁺ reabsorption (thus ↓ ECF volume)

- ↓ Aldosterone production (therefore ↓ Na⁺ reabsorption and ↓ ECF volume).

ASK YOURSELF 4.2 ?

Q1. What are the main contra-indications and common side effects of ACE inhibitors?

Q2.(i) How does diabetic microalbuminuria affect GFR?

(ii) As the course of disease progresses and overt proteinuria gradually reaches nephrotic levels, what change would you expect in GFR?

A1. The main contra-indication for ACE inhibitors is renovascular disease as this can lead to severe hypotension and underperfusion of the kidneys. Two common side effects are significant first dose hypotension and dry cough.

A2.(i) In young adults, the development of diabetic microalbuminuria is usually accompanied by a normal or raised GFR. Older patients with diabetes who develop microalbuminuria may have other risk factors for chronic renal disease and GFR is often already reduced in these patients.

(ii) As renal function deteriorates, the rate of glomerular filtration progressively falls (see Ch. 3).

Glomerular filtration rate

Glomerular filtration rate (GFR) is the product of two factors:

- **Net filtration pressure**

  This represents the sum of the Starling forces:
  - One force contributes to net filtration pressure (i.e. the glomerular capillary hydrostatic pressure)
  - Two forces oppose net filtration (plasma-colloid osmotic pressure and Bowman's capsule hydrostatic pressure)

- **Filtration co-efficient (K_f)**

  The (ultra)filtration co-efficient depends on two specific properties of the (glomerular) filtration membrane:
  - glomerular **surface area** available for filtration
  - glomerular **capillary permeability**.

Thus GFR can be expressed as:

$$\textbf{GFR} \quad = \quad K_f \quad \times \quad \textbf{net filtration pressure} \qquad (4.3)$$

REMEMBER !

Net filtration pressure represents the sum of the Starling forces (each of which is either positive or negative relative to the direction of filtration).

Therefore, GFR may be represented by equation 4.4:

$$\textbf{GFR} \quad = \quad K_f \quad \times \quad (\textbf{P}_\textbf{G} - \textbf{P}_\textbf{B} - \pi_\textbf{G} + \pi_\textbf{B}) \qquad (4.4)$$

K_f = Filtration co-efficient
P_G = Glomerular capillary hydrostatic pressure
P_B = Bowman's capsule hydrostatic pressure
π_G = Plasma-colloid osmotic pressure
π_B = Bowman's capsule colloid osmotic pressure

When calculating GFR mathematically there is another factor to consider, known as the reflection co-efficient (σ) for protein across the glomerular capillary. Since the glomerular ultrafiltrate is virtually protein-free and πB is close to 0, the value of σ is taken as 1. GFR may be expressed as equation 4.4 including σ (see equation below).

$$GFR = K_f [(P_G - P_B) - \sigma(\pi_G - \pi_B)]$$

Fluctuations in the pressures across membranes (i.e. the Starling forces) can result in abnormal body fluid distribution (see *Clinical relevance 4.3*).

Oedema refers to excess accumulation of fluid within the interstitium. In certain pathological states there may be abnormal alterations in the forces that determine movement of fluid across capillary walls i.e. the aforementioned Starling forces. Oedema may be **localised** to a specific region of the body, or **generalised** with disruption of Starling forces across capillary beds throughout the body. Some common causes of oedema are outlined below:

Localised oedema –

- Insect bites/stings cause an increase in capillary permeability (either directly or via inflammatory mediators) and thus ↑ filtration co-efficient, resulting in a rise in filtration rate

- Lymphatic obstruction.

Generalised oedema –

- Compensatory mechanisms in congestive heart failure and physiological changes in pregnancy are common causes of peripheral oedema (feet, ankles and legs)

- Left ventricular failure is associated with pulmonary oedema

- Renal diseases causing nephrotic syndrome (see Ch. 1).

Ascites is the term used to describe free fluid in the peritoneal cavity, presenting as abdominal swelling. The main causes of abdominal distension can be remembered as the **five Fs**: **F**at, **F**aeces, **F**latus (intestinal gas), **F**luid (ascites), **F**etus (in pregnancy).

Approximate concentrations of major solutes in the ultrafiltrate, relative to plasma concentrations:

Plasma [Na$^+$]	=	135 – 145 mmol/L	≈	Ultrafiltrate [Na$^+$]
Plasma [K$^+$]	=	3.5 – 5.0 mmol/L	≈	Ultrafiltrate [K$^+$]
Plasma [Cl$^-$]	=	90 – 105 mmol/L	≈	Ultrafiltrate [Cl$^-$]
Plasma [HCO$_3^-$]	=	22 – 28 mmol/L	≈	Ultrafiltrate [HCO$_3^-$]
Plasma [H$^+$]	=	35 – 45 nmol/L	≈	Ultrafiltrate [H$^+$]
Plasma [glucose] (fasting)	=	4.0 – 6.0 mmol/L	≈	Ultrafiltrate [glucose]
Plasma [protein] (total)	=	60 – 80 g/L	>	Ultrafiltrate [protein]
Plasma [albumin]	=	35 – 55 g/L	>>	Ultrafiltrate [albumin]

Normal laboratory values are provided in Appendix 3.

Renal clearance

The concept of renal clearance arises from the **Fick principle of mass conservation**.

By definition, the value of measured glomerular filtration rate (volume of filtrate produced per unit time and usually expressed in ml/min) should reflect the efficiency of glomerular filtration. Therefore a substance employed in measuring GFR should be freely filterable and must neither be processed by the nephron (reabsorbed or secreted) nor be altered by any physiological process. Renal metabolism of such a substance is described as:

MASS FILTERED = MASS EXCRETED

Furthermore, from a clinical standpoint the chosen substance should not cause harm and must be easy to measure.

In theory, the exogenous high molecular weight carbohydrate inulin (not the hormone insulin!) fulfils these criteria (see *Clinical relevance 4.4*). Inulin can be administered intravenously. Following its distribution throughout the body, and once equilibrium is achieved (equal concentration in the blood plasma and glomerular filtrate) the following measurements are taken, enabling GFR calculation:

Urine concentration of inulin $[U]_{In}$ mmol/ml
Urine flow rate V ml/min
Plasma concentration of inulin $[P]_{In}$ mmol/ml

Inulin clearance rate $=$ $$\frac{[U]_{In} \times V}{[P]_{In}}$$
(measure of GFR)

(4.5)

> **REMEMBER** !
>
> **Units of measure are variable**. In an exam, for example, you may be asked to convert your answers from ml/min to provide the value in L/min or L/d. This is simple enough to do, so always read the question carefully.

ASK YOURSELF 4.3 ?

Q. Given a GFR value of 125 ml/min and daily urine output of 1.5 L, how much fluid is filtered and reabsorbed over a 24 h period?

A. At this GFR, 180 L of fluid is filtered in 24 h. Since normal urine output is only around 1–2 L/d, 99% of the glomerular filtrate is normally reabsorbed into the peritubular capillary network.

Fluid filtered over 24 h:

125 ml = 0.125 L   1h = 60 min
so, 24 h = 24 × 60 = 1440 min
0.125 L × 1440 min = **180 L/d**

Percentage reabsorption:

180 L total filtered load – 1.5 L excretion (urine output)
= 178.5 L reabsorption
(178.5 ÷ 180) × 100 ≈ **99%**

The filtered load calculation is explained in Chapter 5.

CLINICAL RELEVANCE 4.4 ✚

GFR is a **precise measure of renal function** in an individual. However in clinical practice, measuring inulin clearance is considered impractical and is rarely used. Instead, clinicians commonly rely on measurements of the clearance of creatinine, a daily endogenous product predominantly derived from creatine phosphate metabolism within muscle.

Creatinine clearance is based on two measurements:

- a single serum creatinine level
- urine output collections obtained over a period of 24 hours.

Both glomerular filtration and tubular secretion contribute to the excretion of creatinine, but despite this, creatinine clearance calculations produce values reasonably close to that of inulin clearance. Thus creatinine clearance serves as a reliable **estimation of GFR and renal function**. Several factors need to be taken into account:

- Skeletal muscle mass – rate of production of creatinine is dependent on skeletal muscle mass (males tend to have a higher skeletal muscle mass compared to females, thus creatinine levels will be higher in men)

- Age – influences creatinine levels.

For clinical purposes of establishing renal function, serum creatinine is superior to urea because the level of urea is influenced significantly by GFR and by the rate of urea production. Examples of clinical measures of GFR are summarised in *Clinical Relevance 4.5*.

> **REMEMBER** !
>
> It is the value of **creatinine clearance** (not serum creatinine in isolation) that reflects GFR.

CLINICAL RELEVANCE 4.5 ✚

There are three main methods used to practically calculate an **estimated GFR (eGFR)** in a clinical setting:

- Modification of Diet in Renal Disease formula (MDRD)
- Cockcroft & Gault formula
- Creatinine clearance.

Note that each of these methods, outlined below, enables the calculation of an estimated (not absolute) GFR, allowing clinicians to appropriately adjust drug doses for patients with renal impairment.

- *MDRD formula*
  - takes into account plasma/serum creatinine, age, gender, and ethnicity
  - results are expressed against a standard set body surface area of 1.73 m² (normal eGFR ~ 100 mL/min/1.73m²)

- most widely used method for eGFR calculation in the UK

- **Cockcroft & Gault formula**
  - requires serum creatinine, age, gender and weight
  - if the patient is female, the equation result is multiplied by 0.85

- **Creatinine clearance**
  - serum creatinine levels obtained from phlebotomy and 24-h urine collection (urine volume and urine creatinine levels) are needed
  - eGFR = $([U]_{Cr} \times V)/[P]_{Cr}$.

Net filtration pressure is dependent on the Starling forces:

- Glomerular capillary hydrostatic pressure (favours glomerular filtration) $\approx$ 60 mmHg

- Plasma-colloid osmotic pressure (opposes glomerular filtration) $\approx$ 25 mmHg

- Bowman's capsule hydrostatic pressure (opposes glomerular filtration) $\approx$ 15 mmHg

- Bowman's capsule osmotic pressure (negligible).

Hydrostatic pressure depends on the flow of fluid (pressure and resistance).

Colloid-osmotic (oncotic) pressure is due to protein.

Glomerular filtration rate (GFR) is used to gauge renal function. It is the product of the filtration co-efficient factor and net filtration pressure:

$$GFR = K_f \times \text{Net filtration pressure}$$

Any substance meeting the criteria listed below is suitable for measuring GFR:

1. Freely filtered across the filtration barrier into Bowman's space.

2. Neither reabsorbed nor secreted by the nephron.

3. Neither produced nor metabolised by the kidney.

4. Does not directly modify GFR.

5. Inert and harmless, and easily measurable.

In clinical medicine, creatinine measurement is required for the calculation of estimated GFR (eGFR). The use of creatinine has some limitations (see *Clinical Relevance 4.4*).

In a healthy adult male the normal range for GFR is 120–125 ml/min and in females it is approximately 10% less.

Filtration fraction

This is the proportion of plasma entering the glomerulus that is filtered (to form filtrate). Its calculation (see equation 4.6) is based on two values:

- **Glomerular filtration rate (GFR)** – measured by inulin clearance (see *Clinical relevance 4.4*)
- **Renal plasma flow (RPF)** – measured by the clearance rate of the organic anion para-aminohippuric acid (PAH).

$$\frac{\text{Filtration}}{\text{fraction}} = \frac{GFR}{RPF} \qquad (4.6)$$

Renal plasma flow

PAH is freely filtered and is not reabsorbed. However it is different to inulin because any PAH still remaining in the plasma following filtration, is completely secreted into the proximal renal tubule. This is not the case if the transport maximum of PAH is exceeded. This means that plasma PAH is equal to PAH excreted in the urine. Therefore, clearance of PAH (see equation 4.5) is a reasonably accurate estimate of renal plasma flow. This method underestimates the true renal plasma flow by about 10% because blood flow to the kidneys is not restricted to the glomeruli and tubules, but also supplies the peri-renal fat, renal capsule and medulla (see Ch. 3). Renal plasma flow is approximately 600ml/min.

Q. If renal plasma flow falls with a stable GFR, the filtration fraction will increase. What is an important consequence of this, with regard to net filtration pressure?

A. If the fraction of filtered fluid increases, the difference in concentration (i.e. the concentration gradient) of plasma proteins across the membrane will increase. Thus the plasma-colloid osmotic pressure will rise. This potentiates a reduction in GFR because plasma-colloid osmotic pressure opposes net filtration pressure (see *Key points 4.3*).

RENAL BLOOD FLOW

The value of renal blood flow (the vascular supply to the kidneys) can be determined from known values of:

- **Renal plasma flow (RPF)**

- **Packed cell volume (PCV).**

Normal average values for PCV (40%) and RPF (600 ml/min) are used to calculate renal blood flow (RBF) in equation 4.7.

$$\text{Renal blood flow (RBF)} = \frac{\text{RPF}}{1 - \text{PCV}} = \frac{600}{(1 - 0.4)} = \frac{600}{0.6} = \frac{1000}{\text{ml/min}}$$

(4.7)

CLINICAL RELEVANCE 4.6 ✚

Packed cell volume (haematocrit) is the fraction of the total blood volume that is occupied by red cells. So it follows that a raised haematocrit (termed polycythaemia) may be due to:

- ↓ total plasma volume from any cause of dehydration (known as **relative polycythaemia**)

- ↑ total red cell volume (**absolute polycythaemia**).

Absolute polycythaemia can be further defined according to the underlying cause of raised red cell volume:

- **Primary polycythaemia** – intrinsic abnormality of myeloid stem cells

- **Secondary polycythaemia** – increased erythropoietin stimulating erythrocyte (red blood cell) progenitor cells, occurring in response to high altitude, COPD and smoking. Renal carcinoma may be an underlying cause.

Polycythaemia can cause a decrease in renal blood flow. Calculation of haematocrit is useful in detecting polycythaemia clinically (see Ch. 1).

POINTS OF INTEREST 4.6 💭

Polycythaemia is an endocrinopathy sometimes associated with a paraneoplastic syndrome (a constellation of symptoms which may present in patients with malignant disease). Paraneoplastic syndromes are relatively rare but important to recognise.

KEY POINTS 4.4 🔑

Normal average values in a healthy, 70 kg adult:

Filtration fraction (FF) =
Glomerular filtration rate (GFR) ÷ Renal plasma flow (RPF)
Normal average FF ≈ 20%.

Renal blood flow (RBF) = RPF ÷ [1 – Packed cell volume (PCV)]
Normal average RBF ≈ 1000 ml/min (maintained at 20–25% of cardiac output).

The normal range of **PCV** values in healthy adult males is 0.4–0.52 and in females it is 0.36–0.48.
RPF is normally ~ 600 ml/min.

ASK YOURSELF 4.5 ?

Q1. What cardiac output is required to maintain renal blood flow at ~ 1 L/min?

Q2. If the arterial blood pressure fell significantly what would happen to the renal blood flow and thus the GFR, in the absence of any compensatory mechanisms?

A1. Normal cardiac output is approximately 5 L/min at rest and approximately 1/5 of this supplies the kidneys.

A2. Renal blood flow would decrease due to the fall in cardiac output. If all other factors were to remain constant, GFR would decrease in direct correlation to the reduced glomerular capillary blood pressure – glomerular hydrostatic pressure depends on the pressure of and resistance against blood flow (see **Key points 4.3**).

Looking at equations 4.4 and 4.6, you might expect changes in GFR corresponding with alterations in:

- Arterial blood pressure

- Net filtration rate.

However the kidneys are able to maintain a relatively stable GFR and RBF even though arterial pressure varies in response to changes in the external and internal environment (Fig. 4.6). Mechanisms of GFR regulation can be grouped as:

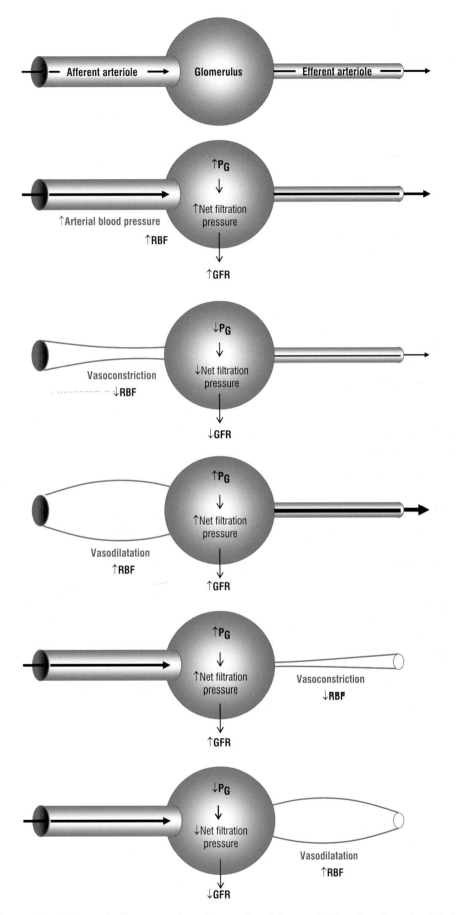

Figure 4.6 – Effects of adjustments in calibre and resistance of either the afferent arteriole or efferent arteriole on RBF and GFR

- **Intrinsic processes of autoregulation** – oppose sudden changes and maintain GFR and RBF at relatively constant levels
- **Extrinsic factors and hormones** – affect GFR and RBF via long-term regulation of arterial blood pressure.

Dysregulation of GFR and RBF is described in *Clinical relevance 4.7*.

Intrinsic mechanisms of autoregulation

Two major mechanisms are believed to contribute to autoregulation:

- **Myogenic** mechanism – detects changes in blood pressure
- **Tubuloglomerular feedback** mechanism – detects changes in the flow of tubular fluid.

These intrinsic mechanisms are described in Table 4.5. Other aspects of the autoregulatory response are yet to be elucidated (see *Points of interest 4.7*).

When considering the regulation of GFR, remember the factors that normally determine GFR can be physiologically controlled (see *Key points 4.3*). The main component of net filtration pressure is the glomerular capillary hydrostatic (blood) pressure, which in turn depends on two aspects of renal blood flow, i.e. the driving pressure (force) and the resistance to flow. The resistance is determined by afferent and efferent arteriolar diameter (see Table 4.3) though the latter is of less importance in the context of autoregulation.

> **REMEMBER** !
>
> The major contribution to autoregulation comes from appropriate adjustments in the diameter of the afferent arteriole.
>
> The efferent arteriole is more important in the context of angiotensin II-mediated vasoconstriction (see Ch. 1) and relative maintenance of GFR.

Each autoregulatory mechanism is considered in turn, when faced with a **rise** in arterial blood pressure:

Myogenic mechanism

The afferent arteriole smooth muscle is stretched, initiating a vasoconstrictive response which increases vascular resistance and counteracts the increased driving pressure, thereby acting to maintain the glomerular capillary hydrostatic pressure within its normal range of 50–60 mmHg.

Tubuloglomerular feedback mechanism

↑ Arterial blood pressure → ↑ Glomerular filtration rate → ↑ Tubular fluid flow rate . . .

At the macula densa in the distal convoluted tubule, cells:

- Monitor NaCl levels in the tubular lumen and detect the change in flow rate
- Respond by stimulating the juxtaglomerular apparatus to release chemicals which have different actions
  - **vasoconstrictive** (e.g. renin release stimulates angiotensin II production)
  - **vasodilatory** (e.g. prostaglandin).

Table 4.5 – Intrinsic mechanisms of autoregulation

Intrinsic mechanisms	
Myogenic mechanism	**Tubuloglomerular feedback mechanism**
Sensitive to changes in **pressure** in the **vascular** system of the nephron	Sensitive to changes in **flow** through the **tubular** system of the nephron
Involves automatic vasoconstriction and dilatation of the **afferent arteriole** in response to stretch and relaxation, respectively.	Involves the **juxtaglomerular apparatus**: Macula densa cells sense changes in fluid flow rate through the tubule and stimulate the release of extrinsic vasoactive chemicals e.g. ATP, NO, prostaglandins

Depending on the balance of vasoactive chemicals and the rate of their secretion, the afferent arteriole either constricts or dilates, maintaining normal flow and glomerular capillary hydrostatic pressure. In response to a rise in arterial pressure, vasoconstriction is required to lower glomerular capillary hydrostatic pressure and maintain normal GFR:

. . . Afferent arteriole constriction $\rightarrow \uparrow$ Resistance $\rightarrow$ $\downarrow$ Blood flow into glomerulus $\rightarrow \downarrow P_G \rightarrow \downarrow$ GFR (see equation 4.4 and Fig. 4.6)

Thus, both intrinsic mechanisms contribute to the maintenance of a normal net filtration pressure and thus restore normal GFR.

CLINICAL RELEVANCE 4.7 ✚

Without autoregulation of renal blood flow, any significant change in mean arterial blood pressure would drastically impact upon urinary excretion (and thus the body's balance) of fluid and electrolytes, resulting in excessive volume depletion or retention.

Sympathetic control may override autoregulation when the mean systemic pressure drops, as occurs in haemorrhage. Compensatory mechanisms, including sympathetic effects on renal vasculature, raise the total peripheral resistance.

ASK YOURSELF 4.6 ?

Q1. If the arterial blood pressure **falls** (as occurs in haemorrhage), consider the role of intrinsic autoregulatory mechanisms, and how the compensatory changes contribute to the body's response to the drop in blood pressure.

Use the grid to structure your answer:

FALL IN ARTERIAL PRESSURE	Myogenic mechanism	Tubuloglomerular feedback mechanism
Detection		
Response		

Q2. Consider the following factors (compensatory changes and their effects) –

i. afferent arteriole diameter
ii. glomerular capillary hydrostatic pressure
iii. net filtration pressure and GFR.

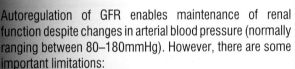

REMEMBER !

Autoregulation of GFR enables maintenance of renal function despite changes in arterial blood pressure (normally ranging between 80–180mmHg). However, there are some important limitations:

- when arterial pressure falls below ~90 mmHg or exceeds the upper limit of normal (i.e. >180 mmHg), the protective autoregulatory mechanisms fail to compensate

- specific neuroendocrine factors may override autoregulation of GFR and RBF.

A1.

FALL IN ARTERIAL PRESSURE	Myogenic mechanism	Tubuloglomerular feedback mechanism
Detection	Relaxation of vascular smooth muscle acts as a stimulant	Macula densa cells in the distal tubule sense the decreased filtrate flow rate due to decreased GFR secondary to the fall in arterial pressure
Response	Reflex vasodilatation	Macula densa cells trigger release of vasoactive chemicals (e.g. prostaglandin) from juxtaglomerular apparatus, promoting vasodilatation

A2.

i. afferent arteriole — Increased afferent arteriole diameter, reducing vascular resistance to flow

ii. glomerular capillary hydrostatic pressure — Increased glomerular blood flow increasing the glomerular capillary hydrostatic pressure

iii. net filtration pressure and GFR — Rise in net filtration pressure and restoration of GFR

'Auto' means 'self', so **auto**regulation is a process of self-regulation. Mechanisms for the autoregulation of blood flow are usually exhibited by body organs sensitive to alterations in their oxygen supply, including the brain and renal tissue. The myogenic mechanism is common to all vascular smooth muscle.

Extrinsic regulatory mechanisms

A number of other factors and hormones play a major role in regulating renal blood flow and GFR, by influencing variables like glomerular hydrostatic pressure and plasma-colloid osmotic pressure. These are the 'extrinsic' feedback control mechanisms, initiated outside the kidneys to effect changes in renal activity (as compared with the aforementioned mechanisms of autoregulation that are intrinsic to the kidneys). The major extrinsic mechanisms are categorised as:

- **Vasoconstrictors**
- **Vasodilators**.

Other regulatory factors are described in *Points of interest 4.8*.

Vasoconstrictors

* Sympathetic control –

Sympathetic nervous system **(adrenergic) fibres** richly innervate renal arteries and arterioles. Under circumstances of normal extracellular fluid (ECF) volume, sympathetic tone remains minimal. A fall in ECF volume increases sympathetic renal drive, with three major effects on renal tubule handling of sodium

ions (Na^+), mediated by different adrenergic receptors (see Ch. 1). Of these effects, increased sympathetic tone acts to decrease GFR and RBF (see Table 4.6).

The effects of anti-diuretic hormone (ADH) are dependent on its concentration:

- At physiological levels – affects collecting duct water permeability (see Ch. 5)
- At high levels – induces generalised vasoconstriction and triggers mesangial cell contraction, reducing the glomerular capillary filtration co-efficient.

*Angiotensin II –

Angiotensin II has a potent vasoconstrictive effect and acts in concert with sympathetic innervation to decrease GFR and RBF. Its release is stimulated by a fall in ECF volume (see Table 4.7).

Endothelin –

Endothelin has a powerful vasoconstrictive effect in pathophysiological conditions, acting to decrease GFR and RBF.

Table 4.8 – Extrinsic regulatory mechanisms: Endothelin (vasoconstrictor)

Endothelin	
Stimuli	Angiotensin II, bradykinin, adrenaline, endothelial shear stress
Secretion sites	Renal vessel endothelium, mesangium, distal tubule
Role in glomerular disease	Vasoconstriction of afferent and efferent arterioles ↓ GFR ↓ RBF

Table 4.6 – Extrinsic regulatory mechanisms: Sympathetic control (vasoconstrictor)

Sympathetic control	Underlying mechanisms	Effects
Afferent and efferent arteriolar vasoconstriction	Vasoconstriction is caused by the binding of noradrenaline (released by sympathetic nerves) and adrenaline (secreted by the adrenal medulla) to α_1 adrenoceptors	↓ GFR (↓ Na^+ filtration)
	A greater constrictive effect on the afferent arteriole (due to the presence of more α_1-adrenoceptors) than on the efferent arteriole, reduces glomerular hydrostatic pressure	↓ RBF
Granular cell renin release	Activation of the Renin-Angiotensin-Aldosterone System (see Ch. 1)	↑ Na^+ reabsorption ADH secretion
NaCl reabsorption	(see Ch. 1)	↑ Na^+ reabsorption

Table 4.7 – Extrinsic regulatory mechanisms: Angiotensin II (vasoconstrictor)

Angiotensin II	Underlying mechanisms	Effect on GFR	Effect on RBF
Low concentration (normal ECF volume)	Disproportionate vasoconstriction: Efferent arteriole > Afferent arteriole. This is due to the greater sensitivity of the efferent arteriole to angiotensin II, compared to the afferent arteriole	↑	↓
High concentration (stimulated by hypovolaemia)	Constriction of both afferent and efferent arterioles	↓	↓

> **REMEMBER** !
>
> The extrinsic mechanisms marked by an asterisk (i.e. sympathetic control and angiotensin II) have differential effects on the afferent and efferent arterioles as described.
>
> If the vasoconstrictive effect is more prominent in the efferent arteriole than in the afferent arteriole there will be a greater effect on the glomerular filtration rate than on renal plasma flow (thus GFR will increase) and vice versa (Fig. 4.6).

Vasodilators

Prostaglandins –

Prostaglandins (PGE_1, PGE_2 and PGI_2) are stimulated by sympathetic activity and act as vasodilators, predominantly affecting the afferent arterioles.

Table 4.9 – Extrinsic regulatory mechanisms: Prostaglandins (vasodilators)

Prostaglandins	
Stimuli	Dehydration, stress, angiotensin II, sympathetic innervation
Secretion	Produced locally within the kidneys
Role	In pathophysiological states: Oppose effects of sympathetic innervation and angiotensin II Limit vasoconstriction to prevent renal ischaemia **↑ RBF** **No change (or ↑) GFR** Ageing: Maintain GFR and RBF

Prostaglandin synthesis-inhibiting drugs and associated renal diseases are described in *Clinical relevance 4.8*.

Nitric oxide –

Nitric oxide (NO) is produced by endothelial cells and its role as a vasodilator is important in maintaining normal renal vessel tone in healthy resting people. It acts to increase GFR and RBF, and its release is stimulated by:

• ↑ **Blood flow**

• **Vasoactive hormones e.g. histamine, bradykinin, acetylcholine**

Bradykinin –

Bradykinin is a vasodilator produced by the enzymatic cleavage of high molecular weight kininogen circulating in plasma. The proteolytic enzyme that catalyses this reaction is kallikrein.

$$Kininogen \xrightarrow{kallikrein} Bradykinin$$

Bradykinin is stimulated by:

• Prostaglandins

• Low levels of ACE

Bradykinin increases GFR and RBF by stimulating:

• Endothelial generation of NO

• Prostaglandins.

Natriuretic peptides –

In hypervolaemic states, natriuretic peptides cause a small increase in GFR with little or no change in RBF, by:

- Dilatation of the afferent arteriole
- Constriction of the efferent arteriole (see Fig. 4.6).

The role of natriuretic peptides in body fluid balance is described in Chapter 1.

Q. How might a disproportionate effect on afferent and efferent arteriole calibre alter the filtration fraction (FF = $^{GFR}/_{RPF}$) ?

A. Greater constriction of the efferent arteriole (relative to the afferent arteriole) causes an increase in GFR and resistance to flow, so RPF decreases (Fig. 4.6). Thus the filtration fraction increases.

Nephropathy associated with Non-Steroidal Anti-Inflammatory Drugs (NSAIDs) –

NSAIDs, like aspirin and ibuprofen, can cause renal damage because the mechanism of drug action involves inhibition of prostaglandin (PGE_2 and PGI_2) synthesis. This reduces RBF and can precipitate renal ischaemia.

Although therapeutic doses of NSAIDs in normal healthy people are unlikely to impair kidney function, NSAIDs are associated with a number of uncommon but important renal syndromes:

- Haemodynamically induced acute renal failure (see Ch. 3)
- Acute drug-induced (or hypersensitivity) interstitial nephritis resulting in acute renal failure with oliguria (abnormally reduced urine output)
    - this is an adverse reaction occurring 2–40 days following exposure to any of a variety of drugs including synthetic penicillins, antibiotics and diuretics
    - interstitial oedema (see Ch. 1) is accompanied by lymphocyte and macrophage infiltration
    - typical features include fever and eosinophilia (a rise in eosinophil count)
    - typical urinary signs include haematuria (blood in urine), mild proteinuria (protein in urine) and leukocyturia (white blood cells present in urine)
    - recognition of the condition and withdrawal of the causative drug results in recovery of renal function
- Minimal change disease resulting in nephrotic syndrome
- Membranous glomerulonephritis with nephrotic syndrome.

Nephrotic syndrome is described in *Clinical relevance 4.9*.

Analgesic nephropathy –

Long-term and excessive use of mixtures of analgesics can have adverse renal effects including chronic renal pathology termed 'analgesic nephropathy', characterised morphologically by:

- Renal papillary necrosis (associated with a number of other conditions including diabetes mellitus)
- Chronic interstitial nephritis.

NSAIDs predispose papillae to ischaemic injury, as described above. Cortical tubulointerstitial nephritis occurs secondary to papillary necrosis. A common complication of analgesic nephropathy is urinary tract infection (see Ch. 3). Other possible clinical features of analgesic nephropathy can be understood by considering the pathological basis of disease:

- Papillary damage leads to **impaired renal concentration of urine**
- Acquired renal tubular acidosis occurring as a consequence of distal tubule damage (see Ch. 2) predisposes to **renal stone development** (see Ch. 3)
- Drug metabolites damage red blood cells, causing **anaemia**.

Other factors that contribute to the regulation of RBF and GFR:

- Adenosine
    - produced locally within the kidneys
    - stimulates vasoconstriction of the afferent arteriole →↓ GFR and ↓ RBF
    - possibly mediates tubuloglomerular feedback

- Adenosine triphosphate (ATP)
    - variable effects on GFR and RBF
    - can cause afferent arteriolar constriction
    - can stimulate NO production

- Histamine
    - released locally
    - acts in healthy resting people
    - acts in states of inflammation and injury
    - reduces arteriolar resistance →↓ RBF with no change in GFR

- Dopamine
  - produced locally in the proximal tubule
  - acts as a vasodilator →↓ RBF
  - inhibits renin secretion.

KEY POINTS 4.5

Afferent arteriole	Efferent arteriole	Resistance to flow	→	RBF	P_G	→	GFR
Constriction –	– Constriction	↑ ↑		↓ ↓	↓ ↑		↓ ↑
Dilatation –	– Dilatation	↓ ↓		↑ ↑	↑ ↓		↑ ↓

Two intrinsic mechanisms of autoregulation maintain relatively constant GFR and RBF by regulating afferent arteriolar tone:

- Myogenic mechanism
  - sensitive to arterial pressure changes
  - intrinsic contraction of vascular smooth muscle in response to stretch stimulus

- Tubuloglomerular feedback mechanism
  - sensitive to changes in tubular fluid [NaCl], detected by macula densa
  - alters afferent arteriolar resistance
  - production and release of ATP by macula densa cells → afferent arteriole vasoconstriction

Major extrinsic regulatory mechanisms for GFR and RBF:

Vasoconstrictors (↓ GFR ↓ RBF)
- Sympathetic nerves
- Angiotensin II
- Endothelin

Vasodilators (↑ GFR ↑ RBF)
- Prostaglandins (modest or no change in GFR) – predominant effect in afferent arterioles
- Nitric oxide
- Bradykinin
- Natriuretic peptides (modest or no change in RBF).

Sympathetic stimulation of the afferent and efferent arterioles may override intrinsic autoregulatory mechanisms.

Efferent arterioles are more sensitive to angiotensin II than afferent renal arterioles.

CLINICAL RELEVANCE 4.9

Glomerulonephritis: Pathophysiology

Many diseases that affect the glomerulus can lead to subsequent renal impairment. **Glomerulonephritis** is the general term used to describe glomerular disease. It can be divided broadly into primary and secondary diseases affecting the glomerulus:

- **Primary glomerulonephritis** – pathology originates in the glomerulus

- **Secondary glomerulonephritis** – consequence of systemic illness.

Common conditions are outlined below.

Primary glomerulonephritis

- *Crescentic glomerulonephritis (Rapidly progressive glomerulonephritis, RPGN) –*

  This is a serious consequence of glomerular damage, with leakage of fibrin and blood into Bowman's space. Stimulation of epithelial cells lining Bowman's capsule to divide, results in the formation of epithelial cell and macrophage **aggregates shaped like crescents in the majority of glomeruli**. This is associated with rapidly progressing renal impairment which, if not quickly treated with immunosuppressive agents, will lead to renal failure.

- *IgA nephropathy (Berger's disease) –*

  Worldwide, Berger's disease is the **most common primary glomerular disease**. It may present after an episode of upper respiratory tract infection. The nephropathy is characterised by **recurrent haematuria and proteinuria**. Microscopy reveals proliferation of, and **prominent IgA deposits in, the mesangium**. There is eventual sclerosis of the damaged segment. Approximately 20–25% of patients develop end-stage renal failure.

- Membranous glomerulonephritis –

  This is **one of the most common causes of nephrotic syndrome in adults**. It is characterised by **uniform, diffuse thickening of glomerular capillary walls**. Immunoglobulin-containing immune complexes (predominantly IgG deposits) form underneath podocytes alongside the basement membrane i.e. the sub-epithelial region. The basement membrane undergoes abnormal changes, thickening around the immune complexes and subsequently becoming pathologically permeable to proteins, resulting in proteinuria. As the disease progresses, excess mesangial matrix (the substance in which mesangial cells are embedded) and glomerular hyalinisation (normal glomerular tissue degenerates into a transparent 'glassy' substance) eventually lead to death of nephrons. The vast majority of cases of membranous glomerulopathy are idiopathic and a small portion are secondary i.e. immune complexes develop because of abnormal antigens e.g. hepatitis or tumour-related (lymphoma).

- *Minimal change disease* –

  This is the **most common cause of nephrotic syndrome in children**. The majority of patients present under the age of 6 years. The primary defect is a **charge imbalance in the glomerular basement membrane (GBM)**. There is no abnormality detected under light microscopy, hence the name 'minimal change'. However electron microscopy reveals widespread fusion of foot processes of podocytes in glomeruli. Prognosis is generally good and **rapid improvement with corticosteroid treatment** is characteristic of minimal change disease.

- *Post-infectious glomerulonephritis* –

  This is typically a diffuse, proliferative glomerulonephritis. The pathology is initiated by an **immune response to exogenous (external) antigen** i.e. the infective organism (e.g. streptococcal, staphylococcal, plasmodial or viral). There is widespread involvement of glomeruli. The main morphological change is **glomerular hypercellularity**.

Secondary glomerulonephritis (systemic diseases with glomerular involvement)

- *Goodpasture's syndrome* –

  This is a rare autoimmune condition characterised by circulating autoantibodies (anti-GBM antibodies) against type IV collagen, a component of pulmonary and glomerular basement membrane. Antibody-mediated injury gives rise to severe and (often rapidly) progressive glomerulonephritis. Consequently, clinical features include lung haemorrhage and renal impairment. Treatment is based on:

  - Removal of the offending autoantibodies by repeated plasma exchange
  - Dampening the inflammatory response with immunosuppressive therapy.

- *Systemic lupus erythematosus (SLE)* –

  This is an inflammatory, multisystem disease of autoimmune origin characterised by widespread vasculitis targeting various organs including the skin, joints, heart, lungs, nervous system and kidneys. Immune complexes that form between immunoglobulins are deposited (resulting in injury) at these organ sites (see *Points of interest*

4.9). Involvement of the glomeruli varies depending on the pattern of glomerulonephritis that develops: membranous, mesangial, focal or diffuse. Clinical features at presentation include haematuria, proteinuria, oedema and hypertension following progression to nephrotic syndrome (see below) or renal failure (see Ch. 3).

- *Diabetes mellitus* – (see *Clinical relevance 4.1*)

- *Amyloidosis* –

  Acquired or inherited systemic disease of abnormal protein folding, in which a pathological proteinaceous substance termed 'amyloid' is deposited extracellularly as insoluble fibrils disrupting normal function. Amyloidosis of the kidney is the most common form of organ involvement.

Glomerulonephritis: Clinical manifestations

Glomerular pathologies can manifest in various ways including haematuria, proteinuria, nephritic syndrome and nephrotic syndrome.

- *Nephritic syndrome* –

  This is a form of partial renal failure with cellular proliferation or division of endothelial cells lining the glomerular capillary lumen, or mesangial cells, because of glomerular damage. The altered histological structure results in:

  - decreased or absent urine output (oliguira or anuria)
  - haematuria
  - failure to excrete nitrogenous waste products like urea (uraemia)
  - fluid retention and hypertension
  - a degree of proteinuria.

  Due to decreased renal perfusion, the Renin-Angiotensin-Aldosterone system is activated resulting in fluid retention and hypertension (see Ch. 1).

- *Nephrotic syndrome* –

  The main features of nephrotic syndrome (massive proteinuria, hypoalbuminaemia, generalised oedema and hyperlipidaemia) are outlined in Table 4.10, alongside the relevant pathophysiological mechanisms.

  In nephrotic syndrome, the damaged 'leaky' filtration barrier allows increased passage of plasma constituents into the renal tubule, resulting in **proteinuria** (and lipiduria). Proteinuria contributes to low plasma albumin, which also undergoes increased metabolic breakdown. **Hypoalbuminaemia** causes body fluid shifts, manifesting as generalised **oedema**. Serum albumin correlates inversely with hypercholesterolaemia, but the cause of the **hyperlipidaemia** is yet to be elucidated.

Table 4.10 – Summary of the characteristic features of nephrotic syndrome

	Nephrotic syndrome
Clinical features	**Underlying pathophysiology**
Heavy proteinuria (loss $\geq$ 3.5g/d)	Initial damage to glomerular basement membrane (GBM) – structural damage and derangement of normal electrical charge permit more and larger molecules to pass through the filtration barrier (described as 'leaky')
Hypoalbuminaemia (plasma albumin < 3g/dL)	$\uparrow$ catabolism of reabsorbed albumin in proximal tubules, Dietary intake of protein increases urinary albumin excretion (through a 'leaky' GBM)
Generalised oedema (see *Clinical relevance 4.3*)	Interstitial oedema is a manifestation of hypoalbuminaemia and nephrotic syndrome, in which renal retention of NaCl and water leads to hypervolaemia increasing glomerular hydrostatic pressure and altering fluid movement across capillary walls
Hyperlipidaemia	Hypoalbuminaemia $\rightarrow \uparrow$ lipoprotein synthesis Proteinuria $\rightarrow \downarrow$ clearance of lipoprotein-bearing triglycerides
Lipiduria	'Leaky' GBM $\rightarrow \uparrow$ lipoprotein filtration (and thus excretion)

REMEMBER **!**

Due to the significant protein loss, individuals with nephrotic syndrome are predisposed to infection (antibody synthesis requires protein!).

POINTS OF INTEREST 4.9

Post-infectious glomerulonephritis represents **exogenous** antigen-induced disease, while an **endogenous** antigen incites the nephritis of SLE.

REMEMBER **!**

The terms 'glomerulonephritis' and 'glomerulopathy' are interchangeable, both referring to glomerular disease.

INTEGRATIVE CASE STUDY

NS is a 12-year-old boy who presents to his physician with a 4 day history of facial swelling, preceded by a mild cold. He is accompanied by his parents who say that apart from mild eczema, NS has always been a healthy child requiring little contact with healthcare professionals.

On examination, the doctor notes significant oedema in the face and around both ankles. On auscultation of the chest, lung fields are clear and cardiovascular examination is normal. Abdominal examination reveals no abnormalities (no evidence of ascites). A urine dipstick test indicates significant proteinuria but no haematuria.

Diagnosis?

- This is likely to be **nephrotic syndrome**.

- The characteristic features of this clinical syndrome include:

  - **heavy proteinuria** (> 3.5g/day, less in children)
  - **hypoalbuminaemia** (< 3g/dL)
  - **generalised oedema** (peri-orbital swelling is typically present)
  - **hyperlipidaemia** and lipiduria.

The underlying pathophysiology is explained in *Clinical relevance 4.9*.

Aetiology?

- There are many causes of nephrotic syndrome. Given this patient's young age, minimal change glomerulonephritis is most likely. This is typically preceded by an upper respiratory tract infection and is commoner in children with atopic conditions (eczema, atopic/IgE-mediated asthma, hay fever).

- Other possible aetiologies to consider include membranoproliferative glomerulonephritis and focal glomerulosclerosis.

Further investigation?

- Blood tests
  - serum urea and creatinine (assessment of renal function, typically normal in nephrotic syndrome)
  - ↓ **serum albumin**

- Urine tests
  - ↑ **24-h urinary protein**
  - microscopic examination of urine

- Creatinine clearance to determine GFR (assessment of renal function)

Management?

- High-dose corticosteroid therapy forms the mainstay of management. Prognosis is generally good, with complete resolution of proteinuria.

✓ **4**

Questions:

The glomerulus

1. Are the following statements **true or false**?

(a) The length and calibre of afferent glomerular arterioles are the same as other arterioles in the body.
(b) Macula densa cells are found in the efferent arteriole endothelium.
(c) Renin is released by granular cells in response to a decrease in Na$^+$ concentration in tubular filtrate.
(d) Angiotensin converting enzyme (ACE) converts angiotensinogen to angiotensin I.
(e) A rise in arterial pressure increases NaCl delivery to the macula densa cells, which act in concert with granular cells to restore normal blood pressure.

Glomerular filtration

2. Are the following statements regarding the filtration pathway and net filtration pressure **true or false**?

(a) The glomerular filtration barrier allows free passage to substances of up to 70 kDa molecular mass.
(b) Plasma proteins pass through the filtration barrier by disrupting the positive charge of the   F
basement membrane. glyco = ⊖ NO   NO
(c) The electrochemical charge of a molecule is the sole determinant of its passage across the filtration barrier. F
                                                                                                                    size

3. Are the following statements regarding glomerular filtration rate and renal clearance **true or false**?

(a) Under normal conditions, plasma-colloid osmotic (oncotic) pressure exerts a greater oppositional force to net filtration pressure than Bowman's capsule hydrostatic pressure.
(b) Normally, glomerular capillary hydrostatic pressure exerts a greater oppositional force to net filtration pressure than the negligible force exerted by Bowman's capsule osmotic pressure.
(c) If glomerular arteriolar resistance remains constant, a change in cardiac output will alter the driving force of glomerular capillary hydrostatic pressure.
(d) The total volume of fluid filtered per day, based on normal values in the average healthy, 70 kg adult, is approximately 180 L. T
(e) In certain pathological states, filtered plasma proteins may appear in Bowman's space, causing an increase in plasma-colloid osmotic pressure. T
(f) The level of serum creatinine in a blood sample is the only measurement required to calculate creatinine clearance. F

Renal blood flow

4. Are the following statements regarding renal blood flow **true or false**?

(a) Vasodilatation of the efferent arteriole does not alter glomerular filtration rate. F
(b) Equal constriction of both afferent and efferent arterioles would not cause a change in glomerular capillary hydrostatic pressure. T
(c) A fall in arterial blood pressure activates intrinsic autoregulatory mechanisms that stimulate vasoconstriction of afferent arterioles, increasing the GFR. dilate F
(d) Angiotensin II has a constrictive effect that predominantly acts on afferent arterioles. F
(e) Normal renal blood flow is approximately 1 L/min (20–25% of cardiac output). T

5. Are the following statements regarding filtration fraction and renal blood flow, based on the values presented **true or false**?

Glomerular filtration rate = 120 ml/min
Renal plasma flow = 600 ml/min
Packed cell volume (haematocrit) = 40%

(a) Based on the values provided, the calculated filtration fraction is 20%. ✓T   20%
(b) Under normal conditions the filtration fraction is usually about 40% in the average healthy, 70 kg adult. F
(c) Based on the values provided, the calculated renal blood flow is 1000 ml/min, which is within the normal range. T

$$\frac{GFR}{RPF} = FF \qquad \frac{120}{600} = \frac{6}{30} = \frac{1}{5} = 0.2$$

CO
↓ 22%
RBF 1.2 L/min
                45%
  ✓55%   ↓
R plasma F   Haematocrit
0.66 L/min

60% = 600ml/min
100% =
0.6 × RBF = 600

Answers:

(see *Key points 4.1*)

1. (a) False. Afferent arterioles in the glomerulus are shorter in length and wider in diameter compared to other arterioles. This contributes to the generation of glomerular hydrostatic pressure.

   (b) False. Macula densa cells are specialised cells in the distal tubule at the juxtaglomerular apparatus.
   (c) True. Renin is released by sympathetic stimulation of granular cells or when the concentration of Na^+ in tubular filtrate (and thus the ECF volume) falls.
   (d) False. ACE converts angiotensin I to angiotensin II.
   (e) True.

(see *Key points 4.2*)

2. (a) True.

   (b) False. The basement membrane contains negatively charged glycoproteins that repel anionic proteins. Plasma proteins and platelets cannot normally pass the filtration barrier.
   (c) False. The charge and molecular size/mass determine the passage of a substance across the filtration barrier.

(see *Key points 4.3*)

3. (a) True.

   Plasma-colloid osmotic pressure ≈ 25 mmHg, Bowman's capsule hydrostatic pressure ≈ 15 mmHg.
   (b) False. Glomerular capillary hydrostatic pressure favours net filtration.
   (c) True. Glomerular capillary hydrostatic pressure is determined by cardiac output and afferent and efferent arteriolar resistance.
   (d) True.
   GFR = 125 ml/min ≈ 180 L/d (1440 min in 24 h).

(see *Ask yourself 4.1* and *Clinical relevance 4.1*)

   (e) False. Plasma-colloid osmotic pressure is determined by the plasma protein concentration gradient.

(see *Clinical relevance 4.4*)

   (f) False. Creatinine clearance is based on two measurements: a single measurement of serum creatinine and 24-h urine collection.

(see *Key points 4.5*)

4. (a) False. Vasodilatation of the efferent arteriole causes a decrease in glomerular capillary hydrostatic pressure (and corresponding decrease in GFR) and an increase in renal blood flow.

   (b) True.
   An isolated increase in afferent arteriolar resistance will decrease glomerular capillary hydrostatic pressure, while vasoconstriction of the efferent arteriole increases glomerular capillary hydrostatic pressure. If two acting forces are equal and opposite, they are said to be in balance and the net effect is nil.
   (c) False. Vasoconstriction of the afferent arteriole decreases the glomerular capillary hydrostatic pressure (less arterial pressure transmitted to glomerulus) thereby reducing the GFR.
   (d) False. Efferent arterioles are more sensitive to the vasoconstrictive effect of angiotensin II.
   (e) True.
   Cardiac output in a normal resting individual is ～5 L/min.

4

✓

(see *Key points 4.4*)

5. (a) True.

    $FF = GFR \div RPF = 120 \div 600 = \textbf{0.2}$.

    (b) False. Normal average FF ≈ 20%.

    (c) True. RBF = 1000 ml/min. The values provided for RPF and PCV are within the normal ranges, so the calculated RBF is within the normal range (20–25% of cardiac output).

    $RBF = RPF \div (1 - PCV) = 600 \div 0.6 = 1000$.

INTRODUCTION TO THE RENAL TUBULE

The renal tubule is the tubular component of the nephron (Fig. 5.1). It begins at the proximal tubule which is a continuation of Bowman's capsule, the initial point of entry for filtered substances. The proximal tubule descends into the renal medulla to become the loop of Henle. This is divided into descending and ascending limbs for descriptive purposes. The ascending limb of the loop of Henle leaves the medullary (inner) region and makes its way towards the cortical (outer) region of the kidney to become the distal convoluted tubule, passing by the juxtaglomerular region of its own nephron. Specialised cells found at this site along the tubule form the macula densa (see Ch. 4). The distal tubule serves as the final site for tubular reabsorption and secretion prior to the emptying of filtrate into the collecting ducts where urine formation is completed. The collecting ducts drain into: renal papillae → minor and major calyces → renal pelvis. Finally urine is transported down the ureters to the bladder where it is stored prior to excretion via the urethra. The organisation of the nephron is described in Chapter 3.

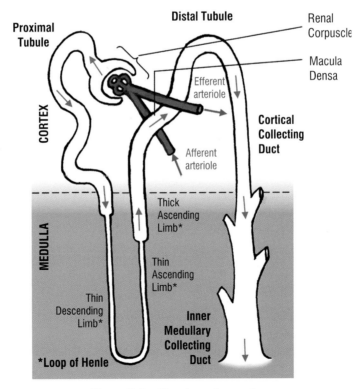

Figure 5.1 – Structure of a nephron

Grey arrows indicate the direction of filtrate flow through the tubular segments.

Four fundamental processes occur along the nephron:

1. **Filtration** – the process by which an essentially protein-free fluid enters the nephron, moving from the glomerular vascular compartment through the filtration barrier to enter Bowman's space (see Ch. 4)

2. **Reabsorption** – the movement of filtered substances from the tubular lumen back into the vascular compartments surrounding the nephron

3. **Secretion** – movement of substances from the vascular compartment to the tubular filtrate

4. **Excretion** – process of eliminating substances from the body. Removal from tubule and out to external environment (via urine).

Each of these terms provides two key pieces of information – where substances are moving from and where they are moving to (see *Key points 5.1*). Descriptions of renal tubular physiology rely on these four terms.

	Intravascular compartment	Nephron	Renal papillae
FILTRATION	Glomerular capillaries	→ Bowman's capsule	
REABSORPTION	Peritubular capillaries	← Tubule	
SECRETION	Peritubular capillaries	→ Tubule	
EXCRETION		Collecting → duct	Urine

The renal tubule is a continuous hollow tube and the 'divisions' are purely descriptive.

The epithelium is one cell layer thick throughout the course of the tubule.

The terms 'filtration', 'reabsorption' and 'secretion' always refer to transfer of substances relative to the blood plasma, unless otherwise specified. Along the nephron, substances are:

- Filtered out of the blood (glomerular capillaries)
- Reabsorbed back into the blood (peritubular capillaries)
- Secreted out of the blood (peritubular capillaries).

Approximately 180 L of ultrafiltrate is produced daily by glomerular filtration, in the average human adult. In the healthy state, ultrafiltrate is essentially free of protein and blood, and contains variable amounts of water, electrolytes and other solutes (e.g. glucose, amino acids, urea and creatinine). Ultrafiltrate is modified by reabsorption and secretion in the tubular system to form urine, which is excreted from the collecting ducts.

POINTS OF INTEREST 5.1

The term 'proximal' refers to a structure that is closer to a point of origin compared to another, while 'distal' describes a structure that is further away from a point of origin. The proximal tubule is near the beginning of the nephron compared to the distal tubule at the far end.

'Convoluted' in the context of the renal tubule describes a segment that is highly or intricately coiled.

KEY POINTS 5.1

The renal tubule is the tubular component of a nephron comprising from beginning to end:

1. Proximal tubule (convoluted and straight sections)

2. Loop of Henle (thin descending limb → thin ascending limb → thick ascending limb/distal straight tubule)

3. Distal convoluted tubule (early and late distal tubule)

4. Collecting ducts

As you go through the listed segments, try to visualise Figure 5.1.

The three cardinal processes in the formation of urine are filtration, reabsorption and secretion. Excretion refers to the removal of tubular fluid from the nephron, in the form of urine.

Tubular transport mechanisms

Cellular transport processes in the renal tubule enable ultrafiltrate modification, which determines:

- The volume and composition of urine
- Fluid and acid-base balance in the intracellular and extracellular compartments.

Transport of solutes across the cell membrane may occur by:

- **Passive mechanisms** – down a chemical concentration gradient or electrical potential difference (i.e. electrical gradient) that does not require metabolic energy
- **Active transport** – against a concentration or electrical gradient, coupled directly to energy derived from metabolic processes, with consumption of adenosine triphosphate (ATP).

Polar molecules and ions are charged and lipophobic, therefore cannot penetrate the lipid bilayer of the plasma membrane. These substances rely on membrane channels and transporters for passage through cells. Movement of substances through open protein channels is a passive process that does not require energy. Important examples are:

- Simple diffusion of ions through membrane protein channels
- Osmosis of water molecules through transmembrane aquaporin (AQP) water channels (see Ch. 3).

Transport mechanisms may be carrier-mediated. Carrier transporters, like channels, are protein components of the cell membrane. However, there are typically more transporters present and they display a higher specificity for the substances they transport, compared to channels.

Active transport requires energy from the hydrolysis of ATP. The Na^+/K^+-ATPase pump is a crucial active transporter in the renal tubule, exchanging every 3 Na^+ ions for 2 K^+ ions. Na^+/K^+-ATPase pumps are located on the basolateral membranes of tubular cells, i.e. the cell surface closest to the basement membrane (see Ch. 3). Na^+ ions leave tubular cells to eventually enter the peritubular capillaries, while K^+ ions are transported from the extracellular environment into tubular cells. Other important active transporters in the kidneys include:

- **Ca^{2+}-ATPase**, for Ca^{2+} reabsorption, predominantly occurring in the proximal tubule and thick ascending limb of the loop of Henle
- **H^+-ATPase and H^+/K^+-ATPase**, for H^+ secretion in the collecting duct system.

Facilitated diffusion of one solute molecule across the cell membrane down its concentration gradient occurs through a uniport mechanism as a passive process. Uniporters play an important role in glucose reabsorption in the proximal tubule, transporting glucose molecules across the basolateral cell membrane into the interstitial fluid.

Facilitated diffusion (passive) and secondary active transport through co-transporters, involve the movement of two or more molecules across the cell membrane. Coupled transport may occur via:

- Symporters, transferring substances in the same direction e.g. Na^+/glucose, Na^+/lactate, Na^+/amino acids, Na^+/PO_4^{3-} transporters located in the proximal convoluted tubule
- Antiporters, e.g. Na^+/H^+ antiport. It is important to note electroneutrality is unchanged and thus maintained when an anion and cation are moved simultaneously by a co-transporter in the same direction, and when solutes of the same charge are transported in the opposite directions by antiporters.

The energy requirement for secondary active transport of an ion against its electrochemical gradient is met through the coupled movement of the other ion down its own electrochemical gradient. For example, in the proximal tubule H^+ ions move through the Na^+/H^+ antiporter against the H^+ electrochemical gradient, driven by the movement of Na^+ down its electrochemical gradient (Fig. 5.3). Thus, secondary active transport of an ion is not directly coupled to ATP hydrolysis.

The different cellular transport processes are summarised below.

Passive mechanisms

Simple diffusion –

- Movement of uncharged solutes across a membrane down their concentration gradient (from a region of higher concentration to one of lower concentration) e.g. O_2, CO_2, fatty acids
- Movement of ions across a membrane down their electrochemical gradient through open protein channels, e.g. Na^+, K^+, Ca^{2+}, Cl^-.

Osmosis –

- Diffusion of water across a membrane down its own concentration gradient through membrane channels, driven by osmotic pressure gradients (see Ch. 1)

- Water that moves across a membrane by osmosis is accompanied by any dissolved solutes, via a process termed 'solvent drag'

- Solvent drag plays a significant role in solute reabsorption in the proximal tubule.

Facilitated diffusion –

- Carrier-mediated transport of specific polar (lipid insoluble) molecules across a membrane down their concentration gradient

- Transport of glucose into cells is the most notable example

- Specific protein carriers in the membrane can become saturated, so facilitated diffusion is limited by a transport maximum

- Different forms of facilitated diffusion are identified:
  - Uniport – movement of a single molecule across the membrane
  - Symport – coupled transport of ≥ 2 molecules in the same direction.

Active transport

Primary active transport –

- Carrier-mediated transport of specific ions or polar (lipid insoluble) molecules across a membrane against their concentration gradient (from a region of lower concentration to one of higher concentration)

- Key examples include Na^+, K^+, amino acids

- Carriers can become saturated, so primary active transport exhibits a transport maximum.

Secondary active transport –

- Co-transport carrier-mediated transport of a specific ion or polar (lipid insoluble) molecule across a membrane against its concentration gradient; this movement is not directly coupled to ATP hydrolysis, but instead is driven by the coupled movement of the other molecule down its own electrochemical gradient

- This is described as an antiport mechanism i.e. coupled transport of ≥ 2 molecules in opposite directions

- Key examples include glucose and amino acids

- Co-transport carriers can become saturated, so secondary active transport exhibits a transport maximum.

Endocytosis –

Invagination of plasma membrane, which surrounds the substance to be ingested and pinches off completely to form an internalised (membrane-enclosed) vesicle in the cytoplasm.

REMEMBER !

Carrier-mediated mechanisms display a transport maximum (T_m). T_m refers to the upper limit of the rate of transfer of a specific substance across a membrane (i.e. the highest rate at which the substance can be moved across the membrane per unit time). Normally the rate of transfer of any substance is related to its concentration. However, when the transport maximum of a substance is reached, all the binding sites are occupied by the substance and the carrier is said to be saturated. Increases in concentration beyond this level do not increase the movement of a substance across a membrane.

Active transport mechanisms that are carrier-mediated move substances across the cell membrane against their concentration gradient. In the case of ions, the ion concentration gradient that drives the transport process is established by the Na^+/K^+-ATPase pump, which is present in the plasma membrane of all cells.

KEY POINTS 5.2

General principles of membrane transport

The terms 'passive transport' and 'active transport' indicate:

- The direction of solute movement relative to its electrochemical gradient

- Whether or not the transport mechanism is directly coupled to metabolic energy

REMEMBER !

The terms 'active' and 'passive' do not tell us whether a transport mechanism occurs through the lipid bilayer, open protein channels or carriers.

Passive transport mechanisms (down electrochemical gradient) –

- Simple diffusion (solutes move through channels)

- Osmosis (water diffuses through channels)

- Facilitated diffusion (carrier-mediated).

Active transport mechanisms (against electrochemical gradient) –

- Primary active transport (carrier-mediated and coupled to ATP hydrolysis) e.g. Na^+/K^+-ATPase

- Secondary active transport (carrier-mediated and driven by electrochemical gradient of coupled ion).

Carrier-mediated mechanisms display a transport maximum, i.e. facilitated diffusion (passive process), primary active transport and secondary active transport.

In the context of coupled transport of ≥ 2 molecules, the terms 'symport' and 'antiport' indicate the direction of movement of a molecule relative to another (the same direction or opposite directions, respectively).

PROXIMAL TUBULE

Functionally, the proximal tubule can be considered in terms of the first half and second half. The initial portion of the proximal tubule is convoluted but straightens prior to its continuation as the descending limb of the loop of Henle (Fig. 5.1). The single-layered epithelium is characterised by cuboidal cells with a densely microvillous lining along the luminal border. This important histological feature increases the surface area available for tubular reabsorption of solutes and water from the filtrate. Adjacent cells are connected to each other via tight junctions found at the luminal border. The cellular ultrastructure is described in detail in Chapter 3.

The proximal tubule is the primary site of reabsorption. For all solutes, this reabsorption is dependent (directly or indirectly) on the action of the Na^+/K^+-ATPase pump, located at the basolateral cell surface.

Sodium

Approximately 65–70% of filtered sodium is reabsorbed in the proximal tubule (Fig. 5.2).

The concentration of sodium within proximal tubule cells is low because of active extrusion of sodium by Na^+/K^+-ATPase at the basolateral membrane (Fig. 5.3). In addition, there is a negative transmembrane potential. Together these factors create a concentration gradient and electrical gradient for luminal Na^+ to move into cells via channels and:

1   Antiporters e.g. Na^+/H^+
2   Co-transporters (symporters) e.g. Na^+/glucose, Na^+/amino acid, Na^+/PO_4^{3-} and Na^+/lactate (Fig. 5.3).

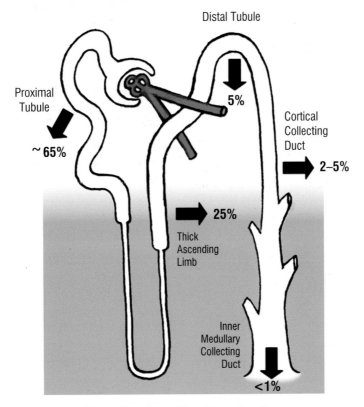

Figure 5.2 – Renal handling of sodium

Distal Tubule

Proximal Tubule

~ 65%

5%

Cortical Collecting Duct

2–5%

25%

Thick Ascending Limb

Inner Medullary Collecting Duct

<1%

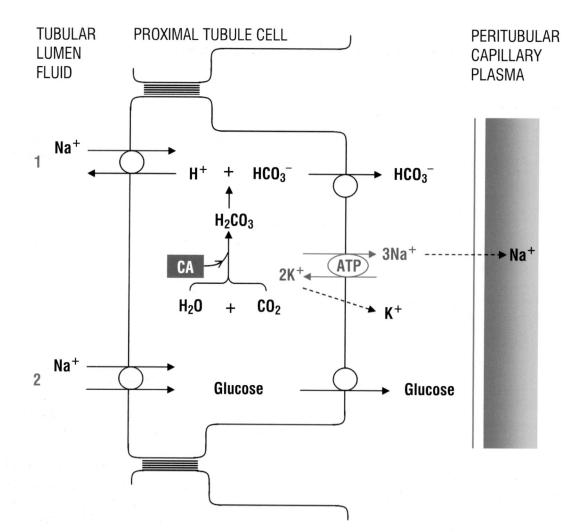

Figure 5.3 – Cellular transport processes in the first half of the proximal tubule

> **REMEMBER** !
>
> In the first half of the proximal tubule, cellular uptake of Na^+ is coupled with H^+ or organic solutes.

> **REMEMBER** !
>
> Reabsorption of other solutes in the filtrate is coupled to Na^+ reabsorption (dependent on Na^+/K^+-ATPase).

In the second half of the proximal tubule, most organic solutes and bicarbonate have already been removed from the filtrate. Therefore sodium leaves the tubular lumen mainly with chloride in the form of NaCl, via two routes described in Chapter 3:

- Transcellular – transport across the luminal membrane via parallel working Na^+/H^+ antiporter and Cl^--base anion antiporters

- Paracellular – diffusion across tight junctions into the lateral intercellular space.

The transcellular route accounts for two thirds of Na^+ reabsorption in the proximal tubule, and the paracellular route accounts for the remaining one third.

Water

The reabsorption of water in the proximal tubule occurs by osmosis through:

- Tight junctions (predominant route)

- AQP water channels at the apical and basolateral cell membranes.

Osmotic reabsorption of water is facilitated by two features of the proximal tubule:

- High water permeability of epithelium

- Osmotic gradient across the tubular epithelium, established by Na^+ reabsorption.

Na$^+$ reabsorption produces an interstitial fluid osmolality that exceeds tubular fluid osmolality. Water moves down its own concentration gradient from the tubular lumen (an area of lower solute concentration) to the intercellular space (an area of higher solute concentration). From the interstitium, water crosses the basement membrane and moves into the peritubular capillaries, also by osmosis. Other physical forces that influence water reabsorption are:

- ↑ **Hydrostatic pressure** in the lateral intercellular spaces – accumulating fluid and solutes due to processes of reabsorption

- ↑ **Plasma-colloid osmotic pressure** in the peritubular capillaries – direct result of glomerular filtration, which removes solutes from the blood at the glomerulus but spares the majority of plasma proteins (thus the concentration of plasma proteins, which determines plasma-colloid osmotic pressure, is relatively high in the peritubular circulation).

The Starling forces are described in Chapter 4.

> **REMEMBER**   !
>
> In the proximal tubule, water reabsorption follows solute reabsorption. This reabsorption is virtually isosmotic, with:
>
> - Reduction in filtrate volume
> - Unchanged filtrate osmolality.

Terms used to describe osmolal concentration are explained in Chapter 1.

Bicarbonate

80% of filtered bicarbonate is reabsorbed in the proximal tubule (Fig. 5.4). Renal tubule handling of bicarbonate (HCO_3^-) is described in Chapter 2.

Na$^+$/H$^+$ antiporters at the apical surface of tubule cells secrete H$^+$ into the tubular lumen, coupled to Na$^+$ transport into cells. H$^+$ enters tubule cells via a reversible reaction with bicarbonate, intermediately forming carbonic acid (H_2CO_3) and subsequently water and carbon dioxide (see equation 5.1). The enzyme involved is carbonic anhydrase (see Ch. 2).

$$H^+ + HCO_3^- \leftrightarrow H_2CO_3 \leftrightarrow H_2O + CO_2 \qquad (5.1)$$

Both H_2O and CO_2 are present at higher concentrations within the tubular lumen than intracellularly. Consequently they enter the tubule cells where the reverse reaction occurs, forming H$^+$ and HCO_3^-. Bicarbonate passes through the basolateral membrane to be reabsorbed into the circulation. The H$^+$ produced intracellularly and secreted into the tubular lumen, is 'reused' by Na$^+$/H$^+$ antiporters and recycled by carbonic anhydrase in this way. The secreted protons are not stagnant and continuously flow with the dynamic filtrate.

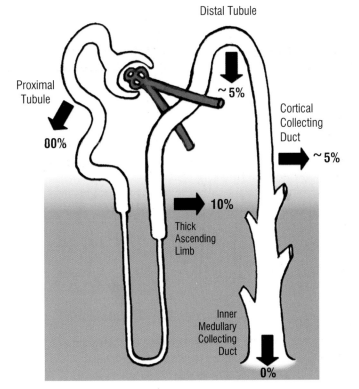

Figure 5.4 – Renal handling of bicarbonate

Chloride

The osmotic gradient in the early part (first half) of the proximal tubule results in greater water reabsorption relative to the reabsorption of chloride ions (Cl⁻). Thus Cl⁻ becomes increasingly concentrated in the filtrate further along the tubule. This creates a Cl⁻ concentration gradient in the second half of the proximal tubule that favours diffusion of Cl⁻ out of the tubular lumen. Chloride ions either enter the interstitium with Na⁺ via tight junctions, or enter the cell via antiporters coupled to another anion, e.g. bicarbonate or formate.

Movement of Cl⁻ (negative charge) out of the tubular lumen establishes a positive transepithelial voltage that favours diffusion of Na⁺ (positive charge) out of the tubular fluid across tight junctions into the blood.

Potassium

Potassium ions (K⁺) are freely filtered at the glomerulus, as are Na⁺ ions (see Ch. 4). However, renal tubule handling of these two ions is very different.

A significant amount of K⁺ (65–70%) is reabsorbed in the proximal tubule (Fig. 5.5). This mainly occurs by passive transport across tight junctions located between adjacent tubular cells. Paracellular K⁺ reabsorption is driven and promoted by:

- The K⁺ concentration gradient established by solvent drag

- Na⁺/K⁺-ATPase action, removing K⁺ from the paracellular space.

> **REMEMBER**   **!**
>
> K⁺ reabsorption is closely linked to proximal tubule reabsorption of Na⁺ and water. Therefore, similar proportions of these three substances are reabsorbed at this site.

Conditions that impair proximal tubule reabsorption of filtrate can adversely affect body fluid and electrolyte balance (*Clinical relevance 5.1*).

CLINICAL RELEVANCE 5.1   ✚

Fanconi Syndrome (De Toni-Fanconi Syndrome)

Proximal tubule reabsorption of filtrate is impaired in Fanconi syndrome. Filtrate contents affected by this rare condition

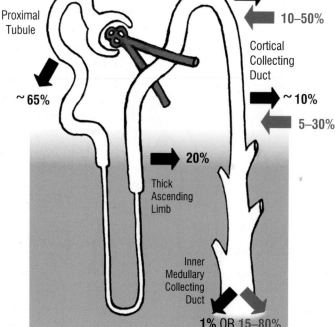

Figure 5.5 – Renal handling of potassium
Black arrows represent reabsorption.
Red arrows indicate secretion.

include phosphate, bicarbonate, glucose, amino acids and uric acid (↑ urinary excretion). If too much bicarbonate is excreted renally, a proximal renal tubular acidosis develops due to the excess of acid resulting from loss of base (see Ch. 2). Fanconi syndrome may be congenital or acquired:

- Congenital Fanconi syndrome – commonest cause is nephropathic cystinosis, where there is impaired metabolism of cystine.

- Acquired Fanconi syndrome – damage to renal tubules by nephrotoxic agents e.g. drugs (expired tetracycline antibiotics) or heavy metals.

KEY POINTS 5.3

Proximal tubule: Sodium handling

The majority of the filtered load of sodium is reabsorbed in the proximal tubule.

Mechanisms of Na^+ reabsorption in the first half of the proximal tubule:

- Membrane channels

- Antiporters e.g. Na^+/H^+

- Co-transporters (symporters) e.g. Na^+/glucose, Na^+/amino acid, Na^+/PO_4^{3-} and Na^+/lactate.

In the second half of the proximal tubule there is a relatively low concentration of organic solutes and HCO_3^-. Na^+ is mainly reabsorbed along this portion with Cl^-, as NaCl:

- Transcellular route ($^2/_3$) – Na^+/H^+ antiporter and Cl^--base anion antiporters

- Paracellular route ($^1/_3$) – diffusion across tight junctions.

Proximal tubule: Water handling

Water reabsorption in the proximal tubule occurs by osmosis, predominantly through tight junctions. The osmotic gradient is dependent on:

- Solute (Na^+) reabsorption

- ↑ Hydrostatic pressure (lateral intercellular spaces)

- ↑ Plasma-colloid osmotic pressure (peritubular capillaries)

Proximal tubule: Bicarbonate handling

The majority of the filtered load of bicarbonate is reabsorbed in the proximal tubule.

HCO_3^- reabsorption occurs via a series of reactions involving the enzyme carbonic anhydrase:

$$H^+ + HCO_3^- \leftrightarrow H_2CO_3 \leftrightarrow H_2O + CO_2$$
$$\text{carbonic anhydrase}$$

The process of HCO_3^- reabsorption (see Ch. 2) relies on Na^+/H^+ antiporters (apical cell membrane).

Proximal tubule: Chloride handling

A Cl^- concentration gradient is created by water reabsorption in the first half of the proximal tubule.

Mechanisms of Cl^- reabsorption in the second half of the proximal tubule:

- Diffusion through tight junctions (with Na^+ as NaCl)

- Antiporters e.g. Cl^-/HCO_3^-.

Proximal tubule: Potassium handling

The majority of the filtered load of potassium is reabsorbed in the proximal tubule, mainly by passive diffusion (paracellular pathway).

LOOP OF HENLE

The loop of Henle is a U-shaped structure in the nephron, involved in urine concentration. It has three main parts continuous with each other: thin descending limb → thin ascending limb → thick ascending limb (also known as the distal straight tubule). The walls of the loop of Henle are lined by squamous cells. Energy-generating mitochondria are found in the cells of the thick ascending limb, driving active processes of Na^+ and Cl^- reabsorption. In comparison, relatively few mitochondria are found in the thin segments of the loop. The cellular ultrastructure of the renal tubule is described in Chapter 3. Potassium ions move in and out of the filtrate along the thin segments of the loop of Henle, resulting in 'recycling' of K^+. A significant proportion of K^+ is reabsorbed at the thick ascending limb.

Different types of nephron are identified:

- Cortical nephron – located in the outer part of the kidney (the cortex) and characterised by a relatively short thin descending limb of the loop of Henle (does not play a significant role in urine concentration)

- Juxtamedullary nephron – located in the transitional region between the outer renal cortex and inner renal medulla, and well suited to its role in the formation of concentrated urine, with a long loop of Henle that reaches the inner depths of the renal medulla (see Ch. 3).

> **REMEMBER**   !
>
> The cortex is the outer part of an organ. Medulla refers to the inner part of an organ.

Table 5.1 provides a summary of solute reabsorption in the loop of Henle. Although each part of the loop of Henle is considered separately in terms of solute handling, it should be remembered that the entire loop is one continuous tube with different functions occurring at specialised sites along the way. This is physiologically significant.

Table 5.1 – Summary of differences in solute handling along the different segments of the loop of Henle

Loop of Henle (segment)	Reabsorption (percentage of filtered substance)				
	NaCl	H_2O	HCO_3^-	Ca^+	K^+
Thin descending limb	–	15% (via AQPs)	–	–	'recycled' across medullary interstitium
Thin ascending limb	25%	–	–	–	
Thick ascending limb	25%	–	10%	20%	20–30%

Thin descending limb

Tubular fluid entering the thin descending limb of the loop of Henle is isotonic, which means the osmolality is equal in the tubular fluid and interstitium. Tubular fluid becomes increasingly concentrated further along this segment by the mechanisms described below, and leaves the thin descending limb with high concentrations of Na^+ and Cl^-. The concepts of osmolality and tonicity are explained in Chapter 1.

> **REMEMBER**   !
>
> The thin descending limb is:
>
> - permeable to water (reabsorption through AQP water channels)
> - impermeable to Na^+.

Reabsorption of water occurs by its passive movement from a relatively dilute solution (tubular fluid in the lumen) to a more solute concentrated solution (hypertonic medullary interstitial fluid). Therefore tubular fluid close to the tip of the loop of Henle is more concentrated than that entering the descending limb at the start of the loop of Henle.

Thin ascending limb

Tubular fluid entering the thin ascending limb is rich in Na^+ and Cl^-, which are reabsorbed passively along this segment by diffusion down the concentration gradient, i.e. from a region of higher NaCl concentration in the tubular fluid to a region of lower NaCl concentration in the interstitium.

> **REMEMBER**   !
>
> The thin ascending limb is:
>
> - permeable to Na^+
> - impermeable to water.

Thick ascending limb

Solute reabsorption across the thick ascending limb occurs via transcellular and paracellular routes:

Transcellular pathway –

- Transcellular reabsorption accounts for 50% of NaCl reabsorption
- Na^+ reabsorption across the apical membrane into the cell occurs via the $Na^+/K^+/2Cl^-$ symporter (NKCC2) and the Na^+/H^+ antiporter

The **$Na^+/K^+/2Cl^-$ symporter** couples the movement of Na^+ and Cl^- down their concentration gradients, releasing potential energy that drives the movement of K^+ into the cell, against its own concentration gradient. A separate K^+ channel in the apical membrane permits movement of K^+ back into the tubule. Potassium ions are 'recycled' in this way, enabling the continued function of the $Na^+/K^+/2Cl^-$ symporter. Dysfunction of the $Na^+/K^+/2Cl^-$ symporter may be pathologically or pharmacologically mediated (see *Clinical relevance 5.2*).

10–15% of filtered bicarbonate is reabsorbed in the thick ascending limb, by mechanisms similar to those in the proximal tubule. This HCO_3^- reabsorption is associated with H^+ secretion (see Ch. 2), which drives Na^+ reabsorption via the Na^+/H^+ antiporter (Fig. 5.6).

This, and the other transport processes described, are driven by the Na^+/K^+-ATPase in the basolateral membrane – the key element driving solute reabsorption in the proximal tubule and thick ascending limb of the loop of Henle.

Movement of these ions out of cells across the basolateral membrane for reabsorption into the blood occurs as follows:

- Na^+ leaves cells through the Na^+/K^+-ATPase pump
- K^+ and Cl^- leave cells through the Cl^- channel (Fig. 5.6)
- HCO_3^- leaves cells by separate pathways (see Ch. 2).

Paracellular pathway –

- Paracellular reabsorption accounts for 50% of NaCl reabsorption
- Passive diffusion of cations (e.g. Na^+, K^+, Ca^{2+}, Mg^{2+}, NH_4^+) from the tubular fluid (Fig. 5.6)
- Driven by the positive luminal charge maintained by transport processes in the apical and basolateral membranes.

> **REMEMBER** !
>
> The thick ascending limb is known as the 'diluting segment'. No reabsorption of water occurs along the entire ascending segment, so the solute reabsorption:
>
> - produces tubular fluid that is dilute (relative to plasma)
> - increases medullary interstitial osmolarity.

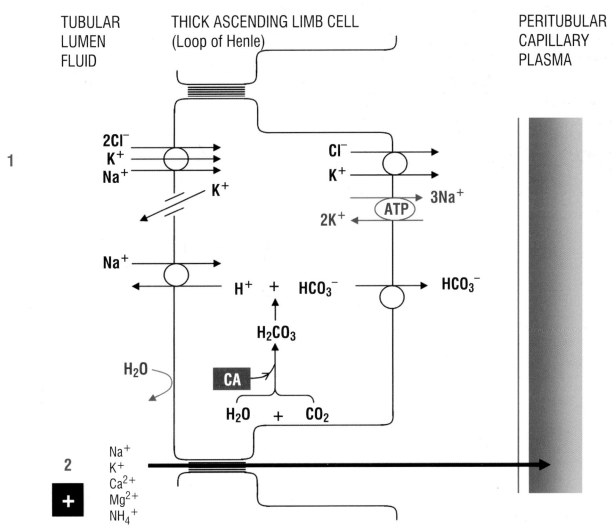

Figure 5.6 – Cellular transport processes in the thick ascending limb of the loop of Henle
The grey arrow indicates water impermeability.

Potassium reabsorption along the thick ascending limb:

1　Is associated with Na^+ reabsorption via the $Na^+/K^+/2Cl^-$ symporter

2　Occurs by the paracellular pathway, favoured by the positive potential in the tubular lumen (Fig. 5.6).

CLINICAL RELEVANCE 5.2 ✚

Thick ascending limb: Pathology

The set of rare autosomal recessive conditions that comprise **Bartter's syndrome** are caused by inherited mutations that impair the activity of the $Na^+/K^+/2Cl^-$ symporter, apical K^+ channel or basolateral Cl^- channel, in the thick ascending limb of the loop of Henle. Due to the inactivation of reabsorptive mechanisms, Bartter's syndrome is characterised by inappropriate urinary excretion of vast amounts of electrolytes (including Na^+, K^+, Cl^-) and water. In response to the resulting hypovolaemia, the Renin-Angiotensin-Aldosterone system is activated to conserve sodium, causing more potassium to be secreted. Consequential hypokalaemia promotes acid secretion, resulting in metabolic alkalosis (see Ch. 2).

Since passive paracellular reabsorption of cations including Ca^{2+}, is dependent on the positive charge of tubular fluid (normally maintained by the transport proteins described above), the dysfunction of these mechanisms results in hypercalciuria (excess urinary excretion of Ca^{2+}) in Bartter's syndrome.

Thick ascending limb: Pharmacology

The thick ascending limb of the loop of Henle is susceptible to pharmacological agents that inhibit ion transport by binding to and blocking the $Na^+/K^+/2Cl^-$ symporter (see Appendix 1). This causes diuresis with the loss of electrolytes that are normally dependent on this transport mechanism for their reabsorption (including Na^+, K^+, Cl^-, Ca^{2+}, Mg^{2+}). Given their site of action, these diuretic drugs are known as **loop diuretics**.

KEY POINTS 5.4 🔑

Loop of Henle

The loop of Henle is considered in terms of three main parts: thin descending limb → thin ascending limb → thick ascending limb.

Thin descending limb:

- Permeable to water (passive reabsorption down osmotic gradient)

- Impermeable to Na^+.

Thin ascending limb:

- Permeable to Na^+

- Impermeable to water.

The properties and arrangement of the thin limbs of the loop of Henle enable K^+ 'recycling' across the medullary interstitium (see *Key points 5.7*).

Thick ascending limb – mechanisms of solute reabsorption driven by basolateral Na^+/K^+-ATPase:

- Transcellular pathway ($\sim$ 50% NaCl reabsorption)
  - $Na^+/K^+/2Cl^-$ symporter
  - Na^+/H^+ antiporter (associated with HCO_3^- reabsorption)
  - Solute reabsorption is not accompanied by water (impermeability of thick ascending limb)

- Paracellular ($\sim$ 50% NaCl reabsorption)

Passive diffusion of cations driven by positive luminal charge.

OTHER MAJOR SOLUTES

Urea

Urea is generated in the liver as a waste product of protein metabolism. Urea is freely filtered at the glomerulus, and its ultrafiltrate concentration equals its plasma concentration. Urea is passively reabsorbed at two sites:

- Proximal tubule (moderate permeability limits this reabsorption to $\sim$ 50% of filtered urea)

- Inner medullary collecting duct (via an ADH-enhanced urea transporter).

All the other tubular segments of the nephron are virtually impermeable to urea.

In the proximal tubule, osmotically induced reabsorption of water exceeds urea reabsorption, with two consequences:

- The concentration of urea in tubular fluid rises along the length of the proximal tubule

- Maintains urea concentration gradient for passive diffusion of urea into the peritubular capillaries.

The urea-rich tubular fluid travels along the nephron to reach the medullary collecting duct, where it diffuses down its concentration gradient into the medullary interstitium. This is where urea accumulates, creating a hyperosmotic medullary interstitium. This hyperosmotic extra-tubular environment is necessary for the maximal concentration of tubular fluid that occurs in the collecting duct, in the final stage of urine formation in the nephron. Movement of urea from the interstitium into the thin descending limb of the loop of Henle through transport proteins also contributes to this process, of recycling urea between the nephron and intersitium.

Phosphate

Over 80% of the body's phosphate (PO_4^{3-}) is found in bones where it plays an important role in metabolism (bone formation and resorption). The remaining 10–20% of PO_4^{3-} is found predominantly in the intracellular fluid, with just under 0.05% located in the extracellular fluid. PO_4^{3-} is an important constituent of organic molecules such as DNA, ATP and intermediate products of metabolism. Urinary PO_4^{3-} is a major constituent of an important buffer system involved in the regulation of acid-base balance (see Ch. 1).

Approximately 85% of plasma PO_4^{3-} is unbound/free and therefore available for filtration at the glomerular filtration barrier. The remaining 10% of total plasma PO_4^{3-} is protein bound and 6% complexed to other ions.

PO_4^{3-} reabsorption sites shown in Figure 5.7 are as follows:

- Proximal tubule (80%)

- Distal tubule (10%)

- Collecting duct (2–3%).

About 80% of the filtered load of PO_4^{3-} is reabsorbed (primarily in the proximal tubule by a transcellular pathway dependent on Na^+ reabsorption) and 10% appears in urine (Fig. 5.7). Na^+/PO_4^{3-} co-transporters are located on the luminal membrane of proximal tubule cells. These symporters transport 2 or $3Na^+$ with each PO_4^{3-}, from the tubular fluid across the apical cell surface to enter tubule cells. PO_4^{3-} leave the basolateral membrane coupled to inorganic anions via antiporters.

Urinary PO_4^{3-} excretion is influenced by several factors including ECF volume, altered serum calcium

levels, dietary PO_4^{3-} intake, chronic changes in plasma pH, and hormones. Of these, the most important is parathyroid hormone, which acts to enhance renal excretion of PO_4^{3-} (see *Points of interest 5.2*).

> **REMEMBER** !
>
> Filtered phosphate that exceeds the maximum rate of reabsorption (limited by T_m) is excreted.

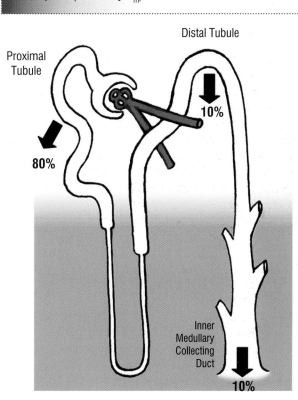

Figure 5.7 – Renal handling of phosphate

Calcium

Almost all the body calcium is stored in bone (~99%), which acts as a source of calcium to replace the ion in situations of low ECF [Ca^{2+}]. Ca^{2+} is involved in many important physiological processes including bone formation, cell division and growth, blood coagulation, muscle contraction and transmission of nerve impulses. Therefore, the maintenance of normal Ca^{2+} distribution within the body is crucial.

Body distribution of Ca^{2+} and PO_4^{3-} is regulated hormonally by parathyroid hormone (PTH), calcitriol and calcitonin. An overview of calcium and phosphate homeostasis is provided in *Points of interest 5.2*.

Unbound/free calcium ions (Ca^{2+}) account for 50% of the total plasma calcium concentration, and are freely

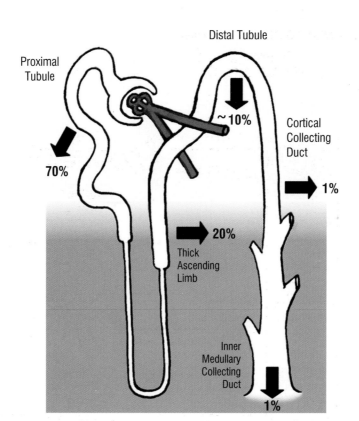

Figure 5.8 – Renal handling of calcium

filtered at the glomerulus. The remaining 45% of the total plasma calcium concentration is protein bound (mainly albumin) and 5% is complexed to anions (e.g. HCO_3^-, citrate, PO_4^{3-}). Plasma pH influences this distribution by altering protein binding to Ca^{2+}.

Filtered calcium is reabsorbed at different sites along the nephron, as shown in Figure 5.8:

- Proximal tubule (70%)

- Cortical portion of thick ascending limb of loop of Henle (20%)

- Distal tubule (5–10%).

Proximal tubule reabsorption of filtered Ca^{2+} occurs via two pathways:

- Paracellular route ($\sim$80%) – passive diffusion across the apical cell surface by solvent drag, and also driven by positive luminal potential in the second half of the proximal tubule

- Transcellular route ($\sim$20%) – movement down electrochemical gradient across Ca^{2+} channels in the apical membrane via calcium-binding proteins, followed by extrusion from cells across basolateral membrane via Ca^{2+}-ATPase.

Ca^{2+} reabsorption in the thick ascending limb occurs by mechanisms similar to those in the proximal tubule, except for solvent drag since the thick ascending limb is impermeable to water. Ca^{2+} reabsorption in the distal tubule is exclusively active and transcellular, under significant hormonal control.

> **REMEMBER** !
>
> The renal threshold is the plasma concentration of a substance at which its T_m is reached, and the substance first starts to appear in the urine. The renal threshold for the inorganic ions PO_4^{3-} and Ca^{2+} is equal to their normal plasma concentrations, which means that the maximal reabsorption of these ions via transport carriers in the renal tubule is equivalent to their normal plasma concentrations. Parathyroid hormone can adjust the renal threshold.

POINTS OF INTEREST 5.2

Homeostasis of these ions depends on two factors:

- Total amount of ion in the body – Ca^{2+} and PO_4^{3-} are absorbed by the gastrointestinal tract and excreted by the kidneys

- Distribution of the ion within the body

  - distribution of Ca^{2+} between bone and ECF

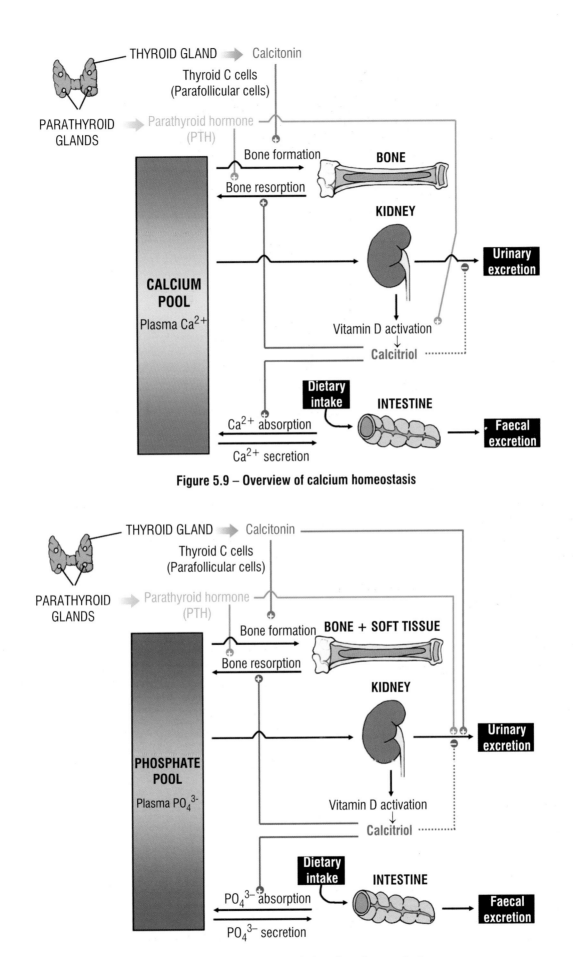

Figure 5.9 – Overview of calcium homeostasis

Figure 5.10 – Overview of phosphate homeostasis

- distribution of PO_4^{3-} between the body fluid compartments of ICF and ECF.

As depicted in Figures 5.9 and 5.10 the distribution of these two ions is regulated by the three hormones listed below:

- **Parathyroid hormone** (PTH), secreted by the parathyroid glands primarily in response to hypocalcaemia i.e. a fall in plasma $[Ca^{2+}]$

- **Calcitriol**, whose metabolism from vitamin D3 is promoted by hypocalcaemia (through its stimulatory effects on PTH release) and by hypophosphataemia i.e. a fall in plasma $[PO_4^{3-}]$.

- **Calcitonin**, primarily secreted in response to hypercalcaemia.

Table 5.2 summarises an integrative review of the role of PTH, calcitriol and calcitonin in the homeostasis of Ca^{2+} and PO_4^{3-}. The net effects of each hormone on plasma levels of Ca^{2+} and PO_4^{3-} are identified.

Magnesium

Unbound/free magnesium ions (Mg^{2+}) are freely filtered at the glomerulus and are passively reabsorbed paracellularly at three sites:

- Proximal tubule (30%) – by solvent drag

- Thick ascending limb (65%) – passive paracellular movement driven by transepithelial potential

- Distal tubule (5%).

Renal tubule handling of Mg^{2+} is influenced by various factors and hormones, outlined in Table 5.3.

Table 5.3 – Summary of hormones and factors affecting renal handling of Mg^{2+}

Factor/Hormone	Effect on renal handling of Mg^{2+}
PTH Calcitonin	↑ paracellular Mg^{2+} reabsorption
Drugs (loop diuretics and thiazides)	↑ Mg^{2+} excretion
Plasma $[Mg^{2+}]$	Ca^{2+}/Mg^{2+} sensing receptor in distal tubule and loop of Henle

Glucose: filtered load calculation

Glucose is an organic molecule of high nutritional importance. Normally, glucose molecules are freely filtered at the glomerulus and almost completely reabsorbed via Na^+/glucose co-transporters in the early part of the proximal convoluted tubule. Thus only minute (usually negligible) amounts may appear in the urine.

> **REMEMBER** !
>
> The Na^+-dependent mechanism of solute reabsorption described above acts to prevent loss of important organic nutrients such as glucose and amino acids.

Key features of glucose reabsorption:

- Secondary active transport – movement of glucose against its concentration gradient from the tubular lumen into cells

- Symport mechanism – transport of glucose is coupled to passive movement of Na^+ across the luminal membrane to enter cells, down Na^+ concentration gradient (maintained by basolateral Na^+/K^+-ATPase)

Table 5.2 – Hormone action at different body sites and net effects on calcium and phosphate ion distribution

	Parathyroid hormone	Calcitriol	Calcitonin
Bone	↑ bone release of Ca^{2+} and PO_4^{3-}	(via PTH action on bone) ↑ bone release of Ca^{2+} and PO_4^{3-}	↓ bone release of Ca^{2+} and PO_4^{3-}
Kidney	↓ kidney excretion of Ca^{2+}	↓ kidney excretion of Ca^{2+} and PO_4^{3-}	↓ kidney excretion of Ca^{2+}
	↑ kidney excretion of PO_4^{3-}		↑ kidney excretion of PO_4^{3-}
Intestine	(via ↑ calcitriol production) ↑ intestine absorption of Ca^{2+} and PO_4^{3-}	↑ intestine absorption of Ca^{2+} and PO_4^{3-}	↑ intestine absorption of Ca^{2+} and PO_4^{3-}
Blood plasma	↑ plasma $[Ca^{2+}]$ ↓ plasma $[PO_4^{3-}]$	↑ plasma $[Ca^{2+}]$ ↑ plasma $[PO_4^{3-}]$	↓ plasma $[Ca^{2+}]$

- Entry into blood from tubule cells – facilitated diffusion of glucose across the basolateral membrane (down its concentration gradient).

REMEMBER   !

Carrier-mediated transport mechanisms exhibit a transport maximum (T_m).

Therefore, all actively reabsorbed substances have a T_m, except for Na^+ (individual Na^+ transport carriers can become saturated but aldosterone up-regulates synthesis of Na^+/K^+ transporters in tubule cells as required).

The transport maximum (T_m) of glucose varies between 300–375 mg/min. If the transporters involved in glucose reabsorption become saturated, less of the filtered load of glucose is removed from the tubular fluid and glucose is consequently excreted in the urine. An acute increase in solute load that exceeds the T_m for that particular solute, cannot be matched by an increase in transporter binding of the solute, and thus limits the rate of its reabsorption.

REMEMBER   !

Filtered load is defined as the quantity of a substance filtered per minute.

Since glucose is freely filtered at the glomerulus, at a constant glomerular filtration rate (GFR) the filtered load of glucose is directly proportional to the plasma glucose concentration (see equation 5.2). The concept of glomerular filtration is explained in Chapter 4.

$$\text{Filtered load of a substance} = \text{Plasma concentration of the substance} \times \text{GFR} \qquad (5.2)$$

The rate of excretion of a substance can be calculated as shown in equation 5.3. This allows calculation of the reabsorption rate, based on known values for filtered load and amount excreted (see equation 5.4).

$$\text{Excretion of a substance} = \text{Urine flow rate} \times \text{Urine concentration of the substance} \qquad (5.3)$$

$$\text{Reabsorption of a substance} = \text{Filtered load of the substance} - \text{Excretion of the substance} \qquad (5.4)$$

ASK YOURSELF 5.1   ?

Q. Using the values provided, calculate:
   (i) Filtered load of glucose
   (ii) Excretion of glucose
   (iii) Reabsorption of glucose

   GFR = 120 ml/min
   Plasma concentration of glucose = 15 mmol/L
   Urine flow rate = 5 ml/min
   Urine concentration of glucose = 120 mmol/L

A. (see equations 5.2–5.4)
   (i) 1.8 mmol/min

   Filtered load = Plasma concentration × GFR
   of glucose   of glucose
                 = 0.015 mmol/ml × 120 ml/min

   (ii) 0.6 mmol/min

   Excretion of = Urine flow × Urine concentration of
   glucose   rate   glucose

               = 5 ml/min × 0.12 mmol/ml

   (iii) 1.2 mmol/min

   Reabsorption = Filtered load − Excretion of
   of glucose   of glucose   glucose

               = 1.8 mmol/min − 0.6 mmol/min

CLINICAL RELEVANCE 5.3   +

Osmotic diuretic drugs (appropriately named after their mechanism of action) e.g. mannitol, can be used to target the proximal tubule and promote the secretion of water. Osmotic diuretics are essentially solutes that remain in the tubular fluid and promote water loss by exerting an osmotic pressure (see Ch. 1). Osmotic diuretics are used in patients with raised intracranial or intraocular pressure.

See Appendix 1.

KEY POINTS 5.5   🔑

Renal tubule handling of other major solutes

Urea:

- Freely filtered at glomerulus

- Passively reabsorbed at proximal tubule and inner medullary collecting duct

- 'Recycling' of urea between tubule and interstitium contributes to concentration of urine (see **Key points 5.7**).

Phosphate:

- Majority of PO_4^{3-} is free for glomerular filtration

- Majority of filtered load of PO_4^{3-} is reabsorbed in the proximal tubule

- Urinary PO_4^{3-} excretion is variable (e.g. influence of PTH).

Calcium:

- ∼50% of plasma Ca^{2+} is free for glomerular filtration.

- Majority of filtered load of Ca^{2+} is reabsorbed in the proximal tubule via

  - Paracellular route (majority)
  - Transcellular route.

Magnesium:

- Majority of filtered load of Mg^{2+} is passively reabsorbed in the thick ascending limb of the loop of Henle, via the paracellular route

- Renal handling of Mg^{2+} is variable (e.g. influence of PTH).

Glucose:

The majority of reabsorption of filtered water, Na^+, Cl^-, K^+ and other solutes occurs in the proximal tubule.

Nearly all the glucose and amino acids filtered by the glomerulus are reabsorbed in the proximal tubule.

Virtually all filtered glucose is reabsorbed, via secondary active transport:

- Na^+/glucose co-transport (apical membrane)

- Passive diffusion (basolateral membrane).

Filtered load calculation:

Filtered load of a substance	=	Plasma concentration of the substance	×	GFR

CLINICAL RELEVANCE 5.4 ➕

Loop diuretics (appropriately named after their site of action i.e. the loop of Henle) e.g. furosemide and bumetanide, prevent

sodium reabsorption by inhibiting $Na^+/K^+/2Cl^-$ symporters in the thick ascending limb thus disrupting the vertical osmotic gradient described above. Increased output of dilute urine is the consequence of administering this class of drug. Loop diuretics are indicated in cases of chronic heart failure and acute left ventricular failure, where excessive accumulation of fluid in body tissues can have serious adverse effects on normal functions and may become life-threatening.

See Appendix 1.

REMEMBER !

Patients with renal impairment (reduced GFR, thus ↓ filtered load of Na^+) may not be as responsive to loop diuretics as healthy patients.

ASK YOURSELF 5.2 ?

Q1. How does a hypertonic solution differ from a hypotonic solution?

Q2. In which part of the loop of Henle (descending limb or ascending limb) would you expect the tubular fluid to be hypotonic and why?

A1. A hypertonic solution is a solution that has a greater osmotic pressure compared to another solution, whereas a hypotonic solution has a weaker osmotic pressure relative to another solution (see Ch. 1).

A2. Tubular fluid is hypotonic as it leaves the thick ascending limb to enter the distal convoluted tubule. This is explained by two features of the thick ascending limb:

- significant solute reabsorption from tubular fluid into the blood

- water impermeability of walls.

DISTAL TUBULE AND COLLECTING DUCT SYSTEM

The distal convoluted tubule is a segment of the nephron that lies entirely within the cortex. It can be divided functionally into two parts: the early distal tubule and the late distal tubule.

Features of the early distal tubule, including specific transport mechanisms that enable solute reabsorption are shown in Figure 5.11 and outlined below:

- Tubular wall impermeable to water

- NaCl entry into cells across the apical Na$^+$/Cl$^-$ symporter, which is inhibited pharmacologically by thiazide diuretics (see *Clinical relevance 5.5*)

- Sodium ions exit cells through basolateral Na$^+$/K$^+$-ATPase activity

- Chloride ions exit cells by diffusion through basolateral Cl$^-$ channels

- Active transcellular Ca^{2+} reabsorption, under hormonal control (Ca^{2+} enters cells through apical Ca^{2+} permeable channels and exits via basolateral 3Na$^+$/Ca^{2+} antiporter mechanism).

CLINICAL RELEVANCE 5.5

Thiazide diuretic drugs (e.g. bendroflumethiazide) target the early distal tubule where they bind to the Cl$^-$-binding site of the Na$^+$/Cl$^-$ symporter, reversibly inhibiting this co-transporter mechanism which is normally responsible for NaCl entry into cells. Administration of thiazide diuretrics is also associated with:

- Decreased Ca^{2+} excretion

- Increased K$^+$ excretion.

Thiazides are effective anti-hypertensives (see Appendix 1).

The collecting ducts can be categorised according to their location within the renal parenchyma, as cortical collecting ducts and medullary collecting ducts. The late distal tubule has similar transport properties to those found in the cortical collecting ducts.

Two characteristic cell types are identified:

- **Principal (P) cells** – responsible for NaCl reabsorption and K$^+$ secretion (both processes dependent on basolateral Na$^+$/K$^+$-ATPase activity)

- **Intercalated (IC) cells** – H$^+$ or HCO$_3^-$ secretion, contributing to the regulation of acid-base balance (see Ch. 2).

Principal (P) cells

P cells reabsorb sodium ions through Na$^+$-selective epithelial channels at the apical membrane. The Na$^+$ electrochemical gradient is dependent on Na$^+$/K$^+$-ATPase activity at the basolateral membrane. The negative lumen potential established by Na$^+$ reabsorption:

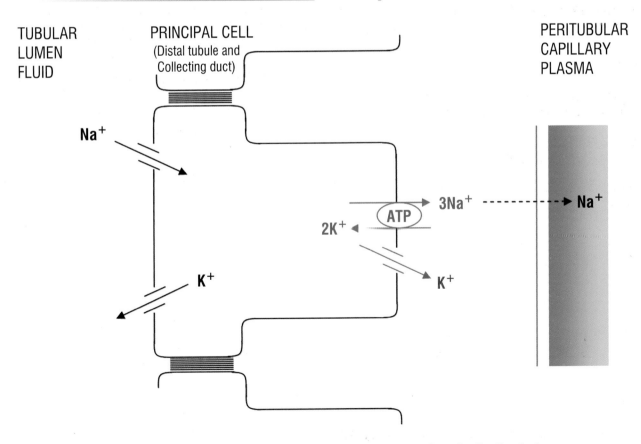

| TUBULAR LUMEN FLUID | PRINCIPAL CELL (Distal tubule and Collecting duct) | PERITUBULAR CAPILLARY PLASMA |

Figure 5.11 – P cell transport processes in the late distal tubule and collecting duct

- Drives paracellular reabsorption of Cl⁻

- Favours K⁺ secretion through apical surface K⁺ channels (at the basolateral membrane, K⁺ continues to enter P cells through Na⁺/K⁺-ATPase activity).

These processes are shown in Figure 5.11.

> **REMEMBER**   **!**
>
> The late distal tubule and collecting duct together form the major site of K⁺ secretion (Fig. 5.5).
>
> Secretion of an ion down its concentration gradient into the tubular lumen is promoted by a high flow rate, which maintains a lower concentration of that ion in the tubular fluid, by 'carrying it away' (osmotic washout).
>
> The relevance of this in the use of diuretics is described in Appendix 1.

The water permeability of the collecting duct system, is mediated by water channels present in P cells (see Ch. 3) promoted by ADH. Therefore water reabsorption across P cells is variable.

Intercalated (IC) cells

Intercalated cells secrete acid into the tubular lumen fluid by mechanisms described in Chapter 2. H⁺-ATPase pumps at the luminal (apical) membrane remove intracellular H⁺ and transport these ions into the tubular lumen. The supply of intracellular H⁺ relies on the reaction between carbon dioxide and water, catalysed by carbonic anhydrase, generating H⁺ and HCO_3^- (see equation 5.1). Bicarbonate ions are removed from IC cells by a Cl^-/HCO_3^- antiporter which transports bicarbonate ions across the basolateral membrane to the interstitium. Various drugs target this segment of the renal tubular system (see **Clinical relevance 5.6**).

IC cells reabsorb K⁺ through H⁺/K⁺-ATPase at the apical membrane, which actively pumps K⁺ into cells.

CLINICAL RELEVANCE 5.6   ✚

Potassium-sparing diuretics target the nephron regions responsible for K⁺ secretion i.e. the late distal tubule and cortical collecting duct (see Appendix 1). These classes of

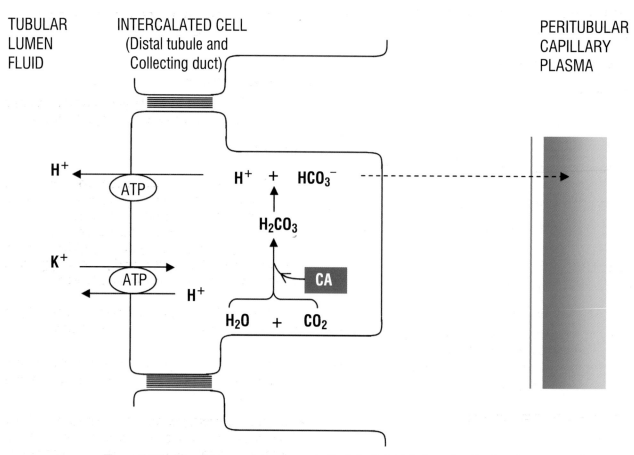

TUBULAR LUMEN FLUID   INTERCALATED CELL (Distal tubule and Collecting duct)   PERITUBULAR CAPILLARY PLASMA

Figure 5.12 – IC cell transport processes in the late distal tubule and collecting duct.

diuretic drugs are considered to be 'K+-sparing' because they act to:

- Inhibit Na+ reabsorption
- ↓ K+ secretion.

This is achieved by two different mechanisms. Thus two classes of K+-sparing diuretics are identified, differentiated by their cellular mechanisms of action:

- Aldosterone receptor antagonists e.g. spironolactone
- Epithelial Na+-selective channel blockers (P cells) e.g. amiloride and triamterene.

In K+ secretion, K+ normally diffuses from the intracellular environment into the tubular lumen down its electrochemical gradient, which is maintained by the charge effects of Na+ reabsorption. If Na+ reabsorption is inhibited (as occurs with these diuretics) the fluid in the tubular lumen becomes more positively charged and the gradient driving K+ secretion is reduced.

REMEMBER !

Aldosterone enhances Na+ reabsorption and K+ secretion by increasing transcription of:

- Epithelial Na+-selective channel
- Na+/K+-ATPase.

KEY POINTS 5.6

The distal convoluted tubule is considered in two parts:

- Early distal tubule
- Late distal tubule (similar features to cortical collecting duct).

Early distal tubule
- Impermeable to water
- Solute reabsorption –
  - Apical membrane transport: Na+/Cl− symporter, active Ca^{2+} transport (transcellular pathway)
  - Basolateral membrane: Na+/K+-ATPase, Cl− channels, 3Na+/Ca^{2+} antiporters.

Late distal tubule and collecting duct
- P cells
  - NaCl reabsorption
  - K+ secretion
  - Dependent on basolateral Na+/K+-ATPase activity

- IC cells
  - H+ or HCO$_3^-$ secretion
  - Acid-base balance (see Ch. 2).

Pathology resulting in damage to tubular epithelium is described in *Clinical relevance 5.7*.

CLINICAL RELEVANCE 5.7 ✚

Acute tubular necrosis (ATN) is a major cause of acute renal failure (see Ch. 3). Two main processes underlie the tubular epithelial cell destruction that is characteristic of ATN:

- Ischaemia due to hypoperfusion
- Direct toxic injury.

Ischaemic ATN –

In **ischaemic ATN**, there is a significant drop in renal perfusion mainly resulting from persistent and severe haemodynamic changes i.e. hypotension and hypovolaemic shock. Hypoperfusion of peritubular capillaries leads to nephron damage. Possible aetiologies of ischaemic ATN include:

- Haemorrhage
- Cardiogenic shock (when the heart fails as a pump, as occurs in cardiac failure)
- Sepsis
- Renal artery stenosis

Ischaemic ATN is characterised by **patchy tubular necrosis with normal 'skip' areas** in between, along the nephron.

Toxic ATN –

Toxic ATN is caused by exposure to nephrotoxic substances that damage tubular epithelial cells. These include exogenous agents (antibiotics e.g. gentamicin or cephalosporins, heavy metals e.g. lead, and others e.g. ethylene glycol) as well as endogenous agents e.g. haemoglobin, myoglobin, bacterial endotoxins. Toxic ATN is characterised by **extensive necrosis, most dramatic in the proximal convoluted tubule**.

ATN can result in imbalances in body water:sodium ratio (see Ch. 1), which vary with different phases of the disease:

- **Acute phase** of ATN – some patients develop **hypernatraemia** believed to be due to renal tubule insensitivity to ADH
- **Recovery (polyuric) phase** of ATN – regeneration of tubular epithelial cells → ↓ plasma concentration of Na+ due to excessive urinary excretion of Na+→ **hyponatraemic dehydration**.

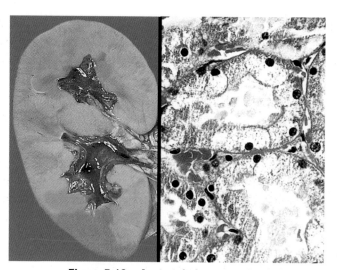

Figure 5.13 – Acute tubular necrosis
Reprinted with permission from Alan Stevens, James Lowe and Ian Scott. Core pathology, 3rd ed. Mosby, Copyright Elsevier (2008).

URINE CONCENTRATION AND DILUTION

The key process in the production of concentrated urine is the reabsorption of water from the hypotonic tubular fluid that flows through the collecting duct. Several mechanisms determine the final concentration of urine. These are outlined below in terms of the counter-current multiplier, vasa recta function, the role of urea, ADH and aldosterone.

Counter-current multiplication

The loop of Henle is the site of the 'counter-current multiplication' effect, primarily because of specific physiological features that act to maintain high medullary osmolality:

Salt must travel 1st now salt! Water always follow

Feature #1 – Water permeability
The ascending limb is impermeable to water but solute reabsorption occurs along this segment. Thus, the ascending limb:

- 'Dilutes' the tubular fluid by the aforementioned transport mechanisms ('single effect' of the counter-current multiplier)

- Contributes to solute accumulation in the medullary interstitium, and thus the high medullary osmolality (this in turn drives water reabsorption along the thin descending limb).

Feature #2 – Solute reabsorption
The thick ascending limb actively extrudes and concentrates solutes into the medullary interstitium by the actions of the $Na^+/K^+/2Cl^-$ co-transporter and Na^+/K^+-ATPase, contributing to the high medullary osmolality.

Feature #3 – Flow of tubular fluid
Flow through the loop of Henle is described as counter-current because it moves in opposite directions through the two parallel limbs of the loop, i.e. the descending limb carries tubular fluid towards the renal medulla, whereas the ascending limb carries tubular fluid away from the medulla towards the renal cortex. This counter-current flow 'multiplies' or amplifies the osmotic gradient between the tubular fluid in the two parallel limbs of the loop.

As a result of counter-current multiplication, the collecting duct is presented with tubular fluid that is hyposmotic (relative to the interstitium). Thus (in the presence of ADH) water diffuses out of the tubular lumen down its concentration gradient. This produces a more concentrated urine. Counter-current multiplication is shown in Figure 5.14.

> **REMEMBER** !
>
> Range of urine osmolality: 50–1400 mOsm/kg H_2O
> Minimum daily urinary excretion of waste products: 600 mOsm/d
>
> Therefore, **minimum daily urine volume: ~ 0.5 L/d**
>
> moles ÷ molarity = volume (see Ch. 1)
> 600 mOsm/d ÷ 1400 mOsm/kg = 0.43 kg/d ≈ 0.5 L/d

Vasa recta function

The vasa recta are capillary networks arising from the efferent arterioles of juxtamedullary nephrons and are the only blood vessels that supply the renal medulla. The vasa recta are paired descending and ascending vessels in parallel with two major functions relating to medullary nephrons:

- Supply of oxygen and nutrients
- Removal of the water and solutes continually added to the medullary interstitium by these nephrons.

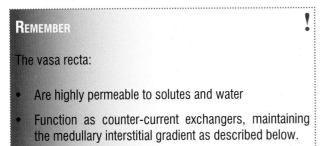

REMEMBER   **!**

The vasa recta:

- Are highly permeable to solutes and water
- Function as counter-current exchangers, maintaining the medullary interstitial gradient as described below.

Water leaves and solutes enter vessels descending into the medulla, while the opposite occurs in the ascending vessels, with no net change in the high medullary interstitial osmolality (see Table 5.4).

Table 5.4 – Summary of water and solute exchange at the vasa recta

	Vasa recta	
	Descending vessels	Ascending vessels
Water	Diffuses out	Diffuses in
Solutes	Enter	Leave

Blood flow through these vessels influences vasa recta function, thus affecting the maintenance of the medullary interstitial gradient:

- ↑ blood flow increases the rate at which osmoles reabsorbed from the medullary interstitium are 'carried away', therefore attenuating the medullary interstitial gradient
- ↓ blood flow decreases the oxygen supply to nephrons, reducing tubular transport activity necessary to maintain the medullary interstitial gradient.

Urea

Renal tubule handling of urea is described earlier in the chapter, in the context of the proximal tubule.

Urea is important in generating a hypertonic medullary environment, acting in conjunction with NaCl. Urea can only permeate the walls of two segments:

- Proximal tubule
- Medullary collecting ducts.

Approximately 50% of filtered urea is reabsorbed in the proximal tubule. As water and other solutes continue to be reabsorbed along the length of the nephron (i.e. segments with low urea permeability – loop of Henle, distal tubule and cortical collecting ducts), the remaining urea becomes increasingly concentrated within the tubule. Thus, at the medullary collecting duct urea leaves the tubular fluid down its concentration gradient to enter the interstitial fluid. In the presence of ADH, this movement of urea is enhanced. 'Recycling' of urea from the interstitium occurs by diffusion of urea into the descending vasa recta to be carried away by the ascending vasa recta to enter the loop of Henle in cortical nephrons. Most of this urea remains within the lumen of the relatively impermeable tubule until the tubular fluid circulates to reach the medullary collecting duct, where urea enters the medullary interstitium once again.

Anti-diuretic hormone

REMEMBER   **!**

Anti-diuretic hormone (ADH) has an 'anti-diuretic' effect, acting to reduce the volume of urine excreted.

The role of ADH in body fluid balance is described in Chapter 1.

ADH is secreted by the posterior pituitary gland in response to a low water balance in the body e.g. following excessive exercise without adequate fluid replacement. Water deprivation manifests as:

- ↑ plasma osmolality
- ↓ ECF plasma volume (blood pressure).

Circulating ADH increases water permeability along the entire length of the collecting duct, by stimulating the integration of existing AQP water channels into the collecting duct luminal/apical membrane. Thus ADH promotes water reabsorption along this nephron segment, in both the renal cortex and medulla. Diabetes insipidus is a condition in which collecting ducts do not respond appropriately to ADH (see *Clinical relevance 5.8*).

ADH increases urea permeability along the final portion of the inner medullary collecting duct. The effect of this is two-fold:

- ↑ urea reabsorption
- ↑ medullary interstitial osmolality.

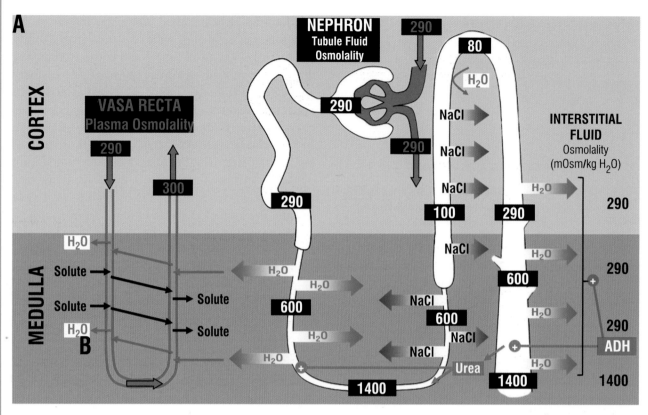

A – Anti-diuresis (excretion of concentrated urine)

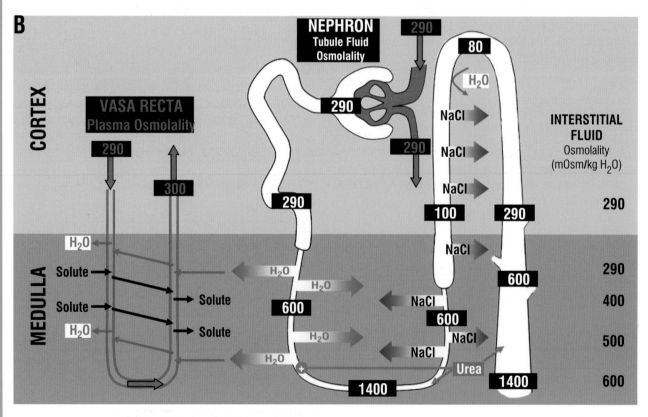

B – Water diuresis (excretion of dilute urine)

Figure 5.14 – Renal tubule dilution and concentration of urine

Curved blue arrow indicates water impermeability of tubule.

ADH also stimulates NaCl reabsorption at the:

- Thick ascending limb of the loop of Henle (may contribute to maintaining the hyperosmotic medullary interstitium)
- Distal tubule
- Cortical collecting duct.

ADH (also known as vasopressin) also binds to receptors on vascular smooth muscle, causing vasoconstriction. This promotes aldosterone-stimulated Na$^+$ reabsorption in the distal tubule.

CLINICAL RELEVANCE 5.8 ✚

Nephrogenic diabetes insipidus is the failure of the kidneys to respond to circulating ADH. Thus water reabsorption in the collecting duct is impaired. This manifests clinically as:

- ↑ production of dilute urine ('polyuria' is the term designated to excessive urination)
- ↑ plasma [Na$^+$] and osmolality → excessive thirst, termed 'polydipsia' (see Ch. 1).

Causes of nephrogenic diabetes insipidus may be:
- Acquired – systemic disorders (e.g. chronic pyelonephritis), lithium therapy, acute tubular necrosis (see *Clinical relevance 5.7*)
- Genetic (rarer) – Inherited mutation of ADH receptor gene or aquaporin channels.

In contrast to nephrogenic diabetes insipidus, in 'central diabetes insipidus' the underlying pathology is ADH deficiency (non-renal aetiology).

Aldosterone

This mineralocorticoid is released by the adrenal glands in response to Renin-Angiotensin-Aldosterone system activation. Aldosterone promotes Na$^+$ reabsorption, mainly in the:

- Distal tubule
- Collecting duct.

As a result, more water is passively reabsorbed in the collecting ducts, and a more concentrated urine is produced.

REMEMBER !

Osmotic water retention as a consequence of Na$^+$ retention, facilitates plasma volume expansion and elevation of arterial blood pressure as part of the body's long-term regulation of ECF volume (reflected by mean arterial blood pressure).

Multiple cellular actions of aldosterone underlie its ability to promote Na$^+$ reabsorption:

- Up-regulation of Na$^+$/Cl$^-$ co-transporter at the luminal (apical) membrane in the early distal tubule
- Up-regulation of Na$^+$-selective epithelial channels at the luminal membrane of principal cells in the late distal tubule and collecting duct
- Na$^+$ cellular entry may also be enhanced in the thick ascending tubule via the Na$^+$/K$^+$/2Cl$^-$ co-transporter
- Up-regulation of Na$^+$/K$^+$-ATPase at the basolateral membrane promotes Na$^+$ extrusion from cells, maintaining the conditions necessary for Na$^+$ reabsorption.

An overview of the Renin-Angiotensin-Aldosterone system is provided in Chapter 1.

REMEMBER !

Urine production is a dynamic process that alters depending on physiological conditions. For example, when the body is dehydrated, the kidneys respond to the increase in plasma osmolality by producing concentrated urine to conserve water. This is dependent on the actions of:

- Loop of Henle (counter-current multiplier effect)
- Vasa recta
- Urea
- Aldosterone
- ADH.

KEY POINTS 5.7 🗝

Urine concentration and dilution

Loop of Henle (Counter-current multiplier):

- Ascending segment – (see *Key points 5.4*)
  - Impermeable to water but solute reabsorption occurs

- Results in dilution of tubular fluid and ↑ medullary interstitial osmolarity

- **Thick ascending limb**
  - Active secretion of solutes (Na$^+$/K$^+$/2Cl$^-$ co-transporter and Na$^+$/K$^+$-ATPase)
  - ↑ Medullary interstitial osmolarity

- Two parallel limbs (descending and ascending) with counter-current flow of tubular fluid.

Vasa recta:

- Capillary networks from efferent arterioles of glomeruli (juxtamedullary nephrons)

- Paired descending and ascending vessels

- Supply medullary nephrons

- High solute and water permeability

- Under normal conditions, maintain high medullary interstitial osmolarity.

Urea:

- ~50% of the filtered load of urea is reabsorbed in the proximal tubule

- Only the proximal tubule and medullary collecting duct are permeable to urea

- Renal handling of urea ('recycling' between the filtrate and medullary interstitium) contributes to the generation of a hypertonic medullary interstitium –
  - Urea passively diffuses down its concentration gradient
    Medullary collecting duct tubular fluid → Medullary interstitial fluid → Descending vasa recta
  - Urea is carried away by the ascending vasa recta
  - Urea diffuses down its concentration gradient
    Ascending vasa recta plasma → Loop of Henle tubular fluid
  - Urea is carried by the impermeable tubule until it reaches the permeable medullary collecting duct, where it again diffuses down its concentration gradient.

Anti-diuretic hormone (ADH):

- Released by posterior pituitary gland, primarily in response to low body water levels

- Reduces the volume of urine excreted (anti-diuresis)

- ADH promotes –
  - Water reabsorption (collecting duct)
  - Urea reabsorption (inner medullary collecting duct)
  - NaCl reabsorption at various tubule sites, including thick ascending limb of the loop of Henle
  - Vasoconstriction.

Aldosterone:

- Stimulated by Renin-Angiotensin-Aldosterone System (see Ch. 1)

- Promotes Na$^+$ reabsorption in the distal tubule and collecting duct, by up-regulating transport mechanisms in different parts of the renal tubule –
  - Na$^+$/Cl$^-$ co-transporters
  - Na$^+$-selective epithelial channels
  - Na$^+$/K$^+$/2Cl$^-$ co-transporters
  - Na$^+$/K$^+$-ATPase at the basolateral membrane

- Osmotic water retention (follows Na$^+$ reabsorption)

- Results in ↑ urine concentration.

CLINICAL RELEVANCE 5.9 ✚

There are essentially two main causes of **tubulointerstitial nephritis**:

- Bacterial infection

- Drug/toxin exposure.

Bacterial Infection –

Bacterial infection of the kidney is known as **pyelonephritis**, one of the most common diseases of the kidney. It can be divided on the basis of acute or chronic infection, differing in aetiology and pathogenesis.

Underlying processes responsible for acute pyelonephritis are outlined below:
- Bacteria (commonly of enteric origin e.g. *E. coli*) can gain access to the lower urinary tract and ascend the ureters (see Ch. 3)

- Septicaemia – haematogenous spread of bacteria to the kidneys via the rich renal vascular supply.

Various factors predispose to acute pyelonephritis:
- Conditions obstructing normal urinary tract flow e.g. enlarged prostate in older men, vesico-ureteric reflux, development of renal calculi (stones), pregnancy, pelvic tumours

- Instrumentation e.g. indwelling urinary catheter (especially long term catheterisation)

- Diabetes mellitus

- Sexual activities

- Compromised immune system e.g. Human Immunodeficiency Virus (HIV)

Chronic pyelonephritis is characterised by widespread fibrosis of renal parenchyma due to chronic inflammation.

Scarring alters the normal pelvi-calyceal structure. There are two forms of chronic pyelonephritis:

- **Reflux nephropathy**

  Reflux of urine through a defunct vesico-ureteric valve causes repeated episodes of tissue inflammation. The condition normally starts asymptomatically in childhood with renal damage becoming obvious in adulthood.

- **Chronic obstructive pyelonephritis**

  Normal drainage of urine is impaired. This predisposes to recurrent infections. Causes of impairment include renal calculi and congenital structural abnormalities.

Drug/Toxin-induced tubulointerstitial nephritis –

Tubulointerstitial damage (inflammation, fibrosis and tubular atrophy) occurs following exposure to an offending agent (NSAIDs, antibiotics e.g. ampicillin, or heavy metals e.g. lead). Long-term analgesia abuse is associated with development of carcinoma in the urinary tract.

Nephropathy associated with analgesic drug exposure is described in Chapter 4.

KEY POINTS 5.8

Renal tubular system: Summary

Tubular transport processes
Various transport mechanisms are seen throughout the renal tubules. Some processes require energy (active transport) while others occur without consumption of metabolic energy (passive transport). Transport mechanisms enable tubular reabsorption of water and solutes, and thus urine production.

Proximal tubule
The majority of solutes and water are reabsorbed at this site in the renal tubules, including glucose.

When the transport maximum (T_m) of glucose is reached, some glucose will appear in urine.

An increase in solute concentration that exceeds the T_m of that solute cannot be matched by an increase in transporter binding of the solute, thus limiting the rate of its reabsorption.

Loop of Henle
There are three different sections:

- Thin descending limb

- Thin ascending limb

- Thick ascending limb.

Juxtamedullary loops of Henle reach deep into the renal medulla and play an important role in producing concentrated urine (counter-current multiplication).

Distal tubule & Collecting duct system
The thick ascending limb of the loop of Henle becomes the distal tubule beyond the juxtaglomerular apparatus. The distal tubule along with the collecting ducts serve as the last sites of tubular filtrate modification prior to urine formation.

These are divided into cortical and medullary collecting ducts.

Two characteristic types of cells with different functions are found in the late distal tubule and cortical collecting ducts:

- Principal cells (P cells) – NaCl reabsorption and K^+ secretion

- Intercalated cells (IC cells) – H^+ or HCO_3^- secretion.

K^+ secretion by P cells is a two-step process:

1. K^+ uptake across basolateral membrane (Na^+/K^+-ATPase)
2. Passive diffusion of K^+ across apical membrane (K^+ channels) down its concentration gradient.

IC cells reabsorb K^+ across the apical membrane via H^+/K^+-ATPase.

Once final filtrate modification occurs, the collecting ducts deliver urine to the ureters via the renal pelvi-calyceal system.

Urine concentration and dilution
The kidneys have the ability to produce both concentrated and dilute urine based on physiological demands. The steep vertical osmolality gradient is a critical aspect of this, and this depends on:

- Counter-current properties of the loop of Henle

- Vasa recta

- Urea

- Secretion of hormones like ADH.

Commonly used anti-hypertensives such as furosemide aim to disrupt this delicate balance and cause polyuria.

REMEMBER !

Na^+ is reabsorbed throughout the nephron, with minimal amounts remaining in the tubular fluid for excretion.

Virtually all filtered K^+ is reabsorbed prior to the filtrate reaching the distal tubule and collecting duct system, where regulated secretion of K^+ occurs, for excretion.

INTEGRATIVE CASE STUDY

AP is a 32-year-old female, 28 weeks pregnant and presenting with general malaise and loin pain. She has a 2 day history of painful and increased frequency of micturition.

On examination, AP is found to be pyrexic (temperature = 39.2°C) and the urine sample appears cloudy and has an offensive smell.

Blood test results:
Serum creatinine = 282 mmol/L   [53 – 106 mmol/L]

Diagnosis?

- This is likely to be **acute pyelonephritis** (bacterial infection of the kidney) following urinary tract infection (UTI).

- UTIs can involve the bladder (cystitis) or the kidneys (pyelonephritis) as in this case.

- Pyelonephritis can be acute or chronic (pathophysiology and predisposing factors are described in *Clinical relevance 5.9*). Patients with acute pyelonephritis typically present with general malaise, loin pain, fever and rigors, ± symptoms of lower UTI. The kidney may be palpable and tender.

- UTIs are very common and groups at higher risk are identified:

    - Congenital abnormalities presenting in infancy: M > F
    - Puberty onwards: F > M due to urethral injury and pregnancy
    - Lower UTI: F > M due to short female urethra.

- Risk factors are similar to those for pyelonephritis (see *Clinical relevance 5.9*).

Further investigation?

Quantitative urine culture is required to establish diagnosis of pyelonephritis.

Management?

- Treatment of UTI and uncomplicated pyelonephritis:

    - high fluid intake
    - regular bladder voiding
    - prophylactic antibiotics

- Important complications of acute pyelonephritis include: renal papillary necrosis, peri-nephric abscess, chronic pyelonephritis, fibrosis and scarring.

- In the case presented, both maternal and fetal health need consideration.

Questions:

The renal tubule

1. Match each segment of nephron to the appropriate function, from the list below.

    i.   Proximal tubule
    ii.   Thin descending limb of the loop of Henle
    iii. Thin ascending limb of the loop of Henle
    iv.   Thick ascending limb of the loop of Henle
    v.   Early distal tubule
    vi.   Late distal tubule and cortical collecting duct
    vii. Inner medullary collecting duct

    (a) Responsible for the majority of reabsorption of the filtered loads of calcium and phosphate. *PCT*
    (b) Impermeable to water, therefore solute reabsorption along this segment has a diluting effect on tubular fluid. *Thick AL*
    (c) Water reabsorption occurs via aquaporin water channels along this Na$^+$-impermeable. segment, producing hyperosmotic tubular fluid associated with dilute urine excretion. *Thin DL*
    (d) The main K$^+$ secretory portion of tubule. *Late DT + CCD*

2. Are the following statements regarding solute handling in the renal tubule **true or false**?

    (a) The largest percentage of the filtered load of sodium is reabsorbed at the proximal tubule. *T 2/3*
    (b) Principal cells are responsible for hydrogen or bicarbonate ion secretion, contributing to the regulation of acid-base balance in the body. *F Int. Cell*
    (c) Potassium ions are reabsorbed across the apical membrane of intercalated cells in the early distal tubule. *F ROMK secretes*
    (d) Hydrogen or bicarbonate ion transport in intercalated cells is dependent on basolateral Na$^+$/K$^+$-ATPase activity. *

3. Are the following statements regarding renal handling of Na$^+$ **true or false**?

    GFR = 180 L/d *≈ 125 ml/min*
    Plasma concentration of Na$^+$ = 137 mmol/L *0.137 mmol/ml*
    Urine flow rate = 5 ml/min
    Urine concentration of Na$^+$ = 240 mmol/L

    1200 → excretion
    $\frac{UV}{P}$ = Clearance
    filtered load

    (a) The filtered load of Na$^+$ is approximately 17 mmol/min. *137 mmol/L ×*
    (b) The expected Na$^+$ excretion is 1.20 mmol/min.
    (c) Almost all of the filtered Na$^+$ is reabsorbed (>90%).

Pharmacology

4. Match the appropriate class of drug to the expected pattern of change in body fluids and/or electrolytes, from the list below. Assume there is no change in diet.

    i.   **Loop diuretic** – self-administered by a healthy body builder for several weeks
    ii.   **Angiotensin converting enzyme (ACE) inhibitor** – for hypertension
    iii. **Thiazide diuretic** – 1 d following administration for hypertension

    (a) ↑ NaCl excretion, ↑ K$^+$ excretion, ↓ Ca^{2+} excretion.
    (b) ↓ urine osmolality, ↑ urine output.
    (c) No change in plasma [Na$^+$], ↓ ECF volume, ↑ plasma K$^+$.

✓ Answers:

(see *Key points 5.1 – 5.6*)

1. (a) i. Proximal tubule.
    (b) iv. Thick ascending limb of the loop of Henle.
    (c) ii. Thin descending limb of the loop of Henle.
    (d) vi. Late distal tubule and cortical collecting duct.

2. (a) True.
    (b) False. Principal cells are involved in NaCl reabsorption and K^+ secretion.
    (c) False. Intercalated cells are located in the late distal tubule and collecting duct, where K^+ reabsorption occurs.
    (d) False. Intercalated cell reabsorption of K^+ is mediated by H^+/K^+-ATPase.

(see *Ask yourself 5.1*)

3. (a) True.

$$\text{Filtered load of } Na^+ \quad = \quad \text{Plasma concentration of } Na^+ \quad \times \quad GFR$$
$$= \quad 0.137 \text{ mmol/ml} \times 125 \text{ ml/min}$$

    (b) True.

$$\text{Excretion of } Na^+ \quad = \quad \text{Urine flow rate} \quad \times \quad \text{Urine concentration of } Na^+$$
$$= \quad 5 \text{ ml/min} \times 0.24 \text{ mmol/ml}$$

    (c) True. Na^+ reabsorption $\approx$ 17 mmol/min.

$$\text{Reabsorption of } Na^+ \quad = \quad \text{Filtered load of } Na^+ \quad - \quad \text{Excretion of } Na^+$$
$$= \quad 17 \text{ mmol/min} - 1.2 \text{ mmol/min}$$
$$= \quad 15.8 \text{ mmol/min}$$

$$\frac{Na^+ \text{ reabsorption}}{\text{Filtered } Na^+} \quad = \quad 0.929 \approx 93\% \text{ (see Fig. 5.2)}$$

4. (see Appendix 1)

(see *Clinical relevance 5.5*)
    (a) iii. Thiazide diuretic.

(see *Clinical relevance 5.4*)
    (b) i. Loop diuretic. The change in urine osmolality is inversely proportional to the change in urine output.

(see Ch. 4)
    (c) ii. ACE inhibitor.

No change in plasma [Na^+] + ↓ ECF volume explained by:
Inhibition of ACE → ↓ NaCl and water reabsorption.

↑ plasma [K^+] explained by:
Inhibition of ACE → ↓ angiotensin II levels → inhibition of aldosterone release → ↓ K^+ secretion by P cells.

APPENDIX 1 - DIURETICS OVERVIEW

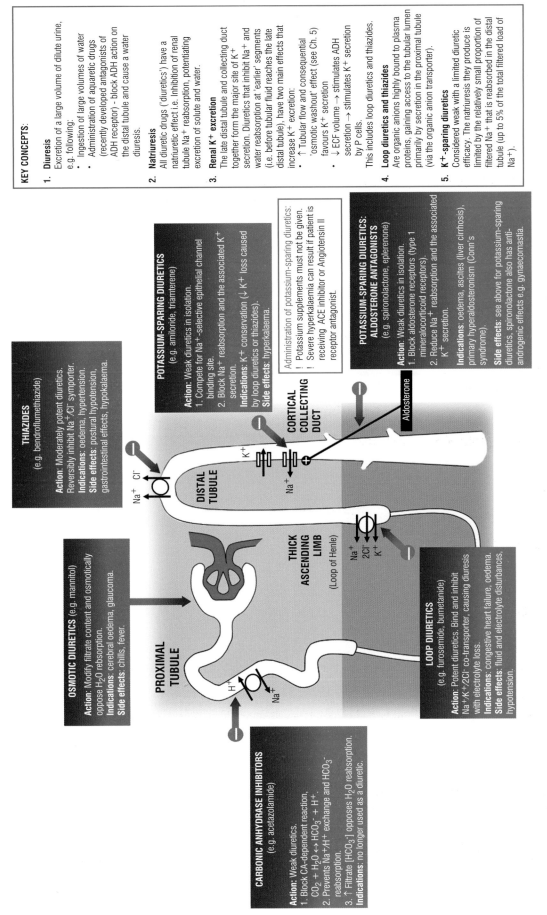

CARBONIC ANHYDRASE INHIBITORS
(e.g. acetazolamide)

Action: Weak diuretics.
1. Block CA-dependent reaction,
   $CO_2 + H_2O \leftrightarrow HCO_3^- + H^+$.
2. Prevents Na^+/H^+ exchange and HCO_3^- reabsorption.
3. ↑ Filtrate [HCO_3^-] opposes H_2O reabsorption.
Indications: no longer used as a diuretic.

OSMOTIC DIURETICS (e.g. mannitol)

Action: Modify filtrate content and osmotically oppose H_2O reabsorption.
Indications: cerebral oedema, glaucoma.
Side effects: chills, fever.

THIAZIDES
(e.g. bendroflumethiazide)

Action: Moderately potent diuretics. Reversibly inhibit Na^+/Cl^- symporter.
Indications: oedema, hypertension.
Side effects: postural hypotension, gastrointestinal effects, hypokalaema.

LOOP DIURETICS
(e.g. furosemide, bumetanide)

Action: Potent diuretics. Bind and inhibit $Na^+/K^+/2Cl^-$ co-transporter, causing diuresis with electrolyte loss.
Indications: congestive heart failure, oedema.
Side effects: fluid and electrolyte disturbances, hypotension.

POTASSIUM-SPARING DIURETICS
(e.g. amiloride, triamterene)

Action: Weak diuretics in isolation.
1. Compete for Na^+-selective epithelial channel binding site.
2. Block Na^+ reabsorption and the associated K^+ secretion.
Indications: K^+ conservation (↓ K^+ loss caused by loop diuretics or thiazides).
Side effects: hyperkalaemia.

Administration of potassium-sparing diuretics:
! Potassium supplements must not be given.
! Severe hyperkalaemia can result if patient is receiving ACE inhibitor or Angiotensin II receptor antagonist.

**POTASSIUM-SPARING DIURETICS:
ALDOSTERONE ANTAGONISTS**
(e.g. spironolactone, eplerenone)

Action: Weak diuretics in isolation.
1. Block aldosterone receptors (type 1 mineralocorticoid receptors).
2. Reduce Na^+ reabsorption and the associated K^+ secretion.
Indications: oedema, ascites (liver cirrhosis), primary hyperaldosteronism (Conn's syndrome).
Side effects: see above for potassium-sparing diuretics, spironolactone also has anti-androgenic effects e.g. gynaecomastia.

PROXIMAL TUBULE

DISTAL TUBULE

THICK ASCENDING LIMB
(Loop of Henle)

CORTICAL COLLECTING DUCT

Aldosterone

H^+ Na^+

Na^+ Cl^-

Na^+ $2Cl^-$ K^+

K^+ Na^+

KEY CONCEPTS:

1. Diuresis
Excretion of a large volume of dilute urine, e.g. following:
- Ingestion of large volumes of water
- Administration of aquaretic drugs (recently developed antagonists of ADH receptor) – block ADH action on the distal tubule and cause a water diuresis.

2. Natriuresis
All diuretic drugs ('diuretics') have a natriuretic effect i.e. Inhibition of renal tubule Na^+ reabsorption, potentiating excretion of solute and water.

3. Renal K^+ excretion
The late distal tubule and collecting duct together form the major site of K^+ secretion. Diuretics that inhibit Na^+ and water reabsorption at 'earlier' segments (i.e. before tubular fluid reaches the late distal tubule), have two main effects that increase K^+ excretion:
- ↑ Tubular flow and consequential 'osmotic washout' effect (see Ch. 5) favours K^+ secretion
- ↓ ECF volume → stimulates ADH secretion → stimulates K^+ secretion by P cells.

This includes loop diuretics and thiazides.

4. Loop diuretics and thiazides
Are organic anions highly bound to plasma proteins, gaining access to the tubular lumen primarily by secretion in the proximal tubule (via the organic anion transporter).

5. K^+-sparing diuretics
Considered weak with a limited diuretic efficacy. The natriuresis they produce is limited by the relatively small proportion of filtered Na^+ that is reabsorbed in the distal tubule (up to 5% of the total filtered load of Na^+).

APPENDIX 2 - CLINICAL IMAGING OVERVIEW

An overview of radiographic anatomy and radiological investigation of the kidneys and urinary tract is provided. Different imaging methods are outlined below with clinical images accompanied by examples of reported findings. Ultrasonography and computed tomography are modalities of first choice in renal imaging. Magnetic resonance imaging (MRI) is useful for differentiating between soft tissues, and its role in assessing renal lesions is developing.

A   Ultrasound (US) Abdomen

Ultrasonography is a non-invasive, non-ionising and relatively quick procedure that uses high-frequency sound waves for the visualisation and evaluation of the size, shape and location of the kidneys and related structures. Renal blood flow may be assessed using Doppler ultrasound. Factors that may interfere with ultrasound image quality include obesity and intestinal gas.

Ultrasonography is useful for assessing:

- Renal cysts – appear as hypoechoic (dark), fluid-filled region

- Tumours

- Abscesses

- Outflow tract obstruction e.g. calculi
    - Dilatation of proximal renal pelvis
    - The stone itself may be visualised (dense structures have an echogenic/echobright appearance, reflecting the ultrasound waves and usually creating an acoustic shadow).

- Collections of fluid

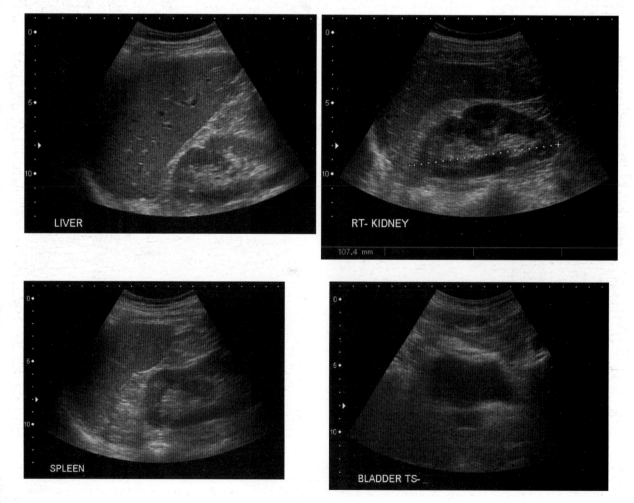

Normal appearances of both kidneys. Prominent column of Bertin noted in left kidney (normal variant – septum of Bertin is an invagination of renal cortex down to the renal sinus, occurring at the junctions of original fetal kidney lobulations). Urinary bladder partially distended but normal in outline.

B   Intravenous Urography (IVU)

These contrast X-ray studies enable visualisation of the kidneys and ureters after the injection of a contrast dye that enhances the image on X-ray film. Contrast medium is injected intravenously and is excreted by the kidneys. X-rays taken at short intervals allow the movement of contrast through the urinary system to be assessed. IVU is often useful in identifying ureteric calculi which obstruct and thus delay the flow of contrast. IVU may be requested in cases where the clinical history and features are suggestive of renal colic (see Ch. 3). IVU may also be useful in assessing renal trauma and tumours.

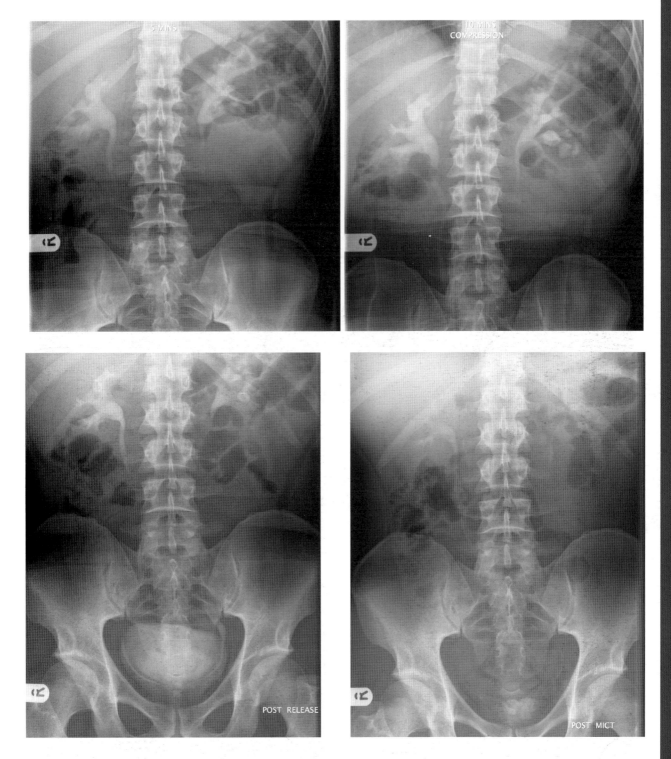

Both kidneys are normal in size, shape and outline. Prompt bilateral excretion. Both pelvi-calyceal systems appear normal. Contrast passes freely down both ureters which are of normal calibre, to the urinary bladder. The bladder is smooth-walled and empties satisfactorily with only a very small residual volume in the post-micturition film (labelled 'POST MICT'). Note the course of the ureters in relation to the tips of the transverse processes of the lumbar vertebrae.

C   Computed Tomography (CT)

This imaging modality combines X-rays and computer technology to generate detailed cross-sectional images of the body ('slices'). This involves the use of a rotating X-ray source and detector, with a moving patient bed.

CT is more accurate than IVU in diagnosing and locating renal tumours and trauma-related lesions. A plain CT scan may be preferable in cases of renal colic and when a patient is unlikely to tolerate intravenous contrast. This imaging procedure is useful in detecting:

- Tumours
- Obstructive conditions
- Congenital abnormalities
- Polycystic kidney disease (see Ch. 3)
- Collections of fluid
- Abscess formation.

CT scans also show other structural abnormalities and pathologies which mimic renal colic and may be missed on IVU e.g. aortic aneurysm.

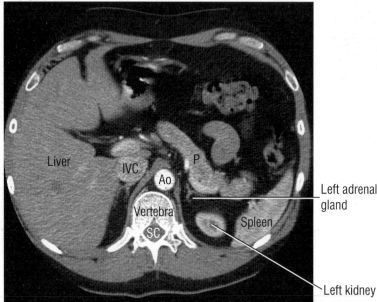

CT scan with contrast – transverse sections

Ao = Aorta
IVC = Inferior Vena Cava
P = Pancreas
SC = Spinal cord

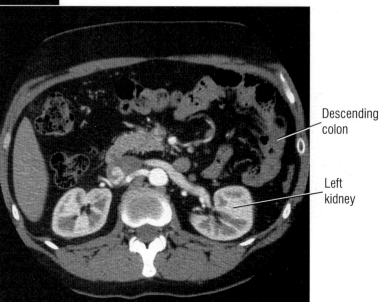

CT scan without contrast – coronal section (left) and transverse section (right)

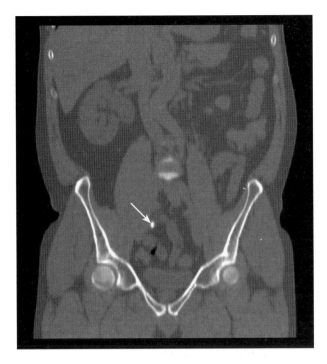

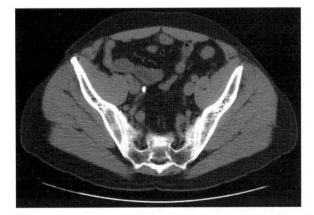

Right kidney demonstrates mild hydronephrosis with dilatation of the right ureter. There is a ureteric calculus at the level of the right sacroiliac joint, obstructing the distal portion of the right ureter. The stone appears as a dense white opacity (arrowed).

D   Micturating Cystourethrography (MCUG)

In this procedure the bladder is filled with contrast through a urethral catheter and views are obtained on voiding. MCUG is normally a paediatric procedure used to demonstrate:

- Vesico-ureteric reflux in recurrent UTI (see Ch. 3)

- Urethral valves or obstruction

- Stress incontinence

- Bladder dysfunctions.

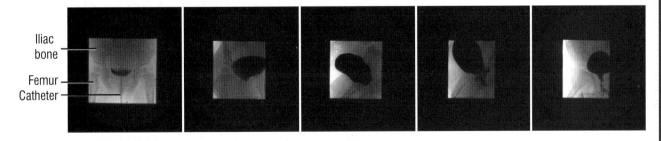

Normal anatomy of the bladder. Normal appearances on voiding. No evidence of reflux during the study.

E   Nuclear Medicine Renography (functional scanning)

While the aforementioned imaging modalities allow assessment of structural features, renal nuclear medicine scans primarily reveal how the kidneys are functioning. There are two types of nuclear medicine renogram, which involve the injection of a radiopharmaceutical (isotope-labelled substance):

- Static scan (using DMSA) – shows functional renal tissue and is primarily used to detect renal scarring (bilateral scarring predisposes to hypertension and chronic renal failure in later life) and to measure differential renal function between the two kidneys

- Dynamic scan (using MAG3) – provides information on blood flow, renal function and drainage.

APPENDIX 3 – NORMAL VALUES

Normal values given are for adults and may vary between laboratories.

Haematology

Haemoglobin	
Male	13.5 – 17.5 g/dL
Female	11.5 – 16.5 g/dL
Mean corpuscular volume (MCV)	80 – 96 fL
Packed cell volume (Haematocrit)	
Male	0.42 – 0.53
Female	0.36 – 0.45
White cell count (WCC)	$4 – 11 \times 10^9$ cells/L
Platelet count	$150 – 400 \times 10^9$ /L
Erythrocyte sedimentation rate (ESR)	0 – 20 mm/h

Arterial blood gases

pH	7.35 – 7.45
PCO_2	4.4 – 5.9 kPa
PO_2	10.0 – 14.0 kPa
$[H^+]$	36 – 44 nmol/L
$[HCO_3^-]$	22 – 28 mmol/L
BE	-2 – +2 mmol/L

Biochemistry

Albumin	35 – 55 g/L
Bicarbonate	22 – 28 mmol/L
Calcium	2.1 – 2.6 mmol/L
Chloride	90 – 105 mmol/L
Cholesterol	< 5.2 mmol/L
Creatinine	60 – 120 μmol/L
Glucose (fasting)	4.0 – 6.0 mmol/L
Magnesium	0.7 – 1.0 mmol/L
Osmolality	285 – 295 mOsm/kg
Phosphate	0.8 – 1.5 mmol/L
Potassium	3.5 – 5.0 mmol/L
Protein (total)	60 – 80 g/L
Sodium	135 – 145 mmol/L
Triglycerides	< 2.0 mmol/L
Urate	0.2 – 0.4 mmol/L
Urea	2.5 – 6.7 mmol/L

COMMONLY USED ABBREVIATIONS

ABG	Arterial blood gas
ACE	Angiotensin converting enzyme
ACTH	Adrenocorticotrophic hormone
ADH	Anti-diuretic hormone
ANP	Atrial natriuretic peptide
AQP	Aquaporin
ATN	Acute tubular necrosis
ATP	Adenosine triphosphate
BNP	Brain natriuretic peptide
BP	Blood pressure
CA	Carbonic anhydrase
cGMP	Cyclic guanosine monophosphate
DKA	Diabetic ketoacidosis
DM	Diabetes mellitus
ECF	Extracellular fluid
ECG	Electrocardiogram
eGFR	Estimated glomerular filtration rate
FBC	Full blood count
FF	Filtration fraction
GBM	Glomerular basement membrane
GFR	Glomerular filtration rate
HIV	Human immunodeficiency virus
ICF	Intracellular fluid
Ig	Immunoglobulin
IVC	Inferior vena cava
MCV	Mean corpuscular volume
NO	Nitric oxide
NSAID	Non-steroidal anti-inflammatory drug
PCO_2	Partial pressure of carbon dioxide
PCV	Packed cell volume
PG	Prostaglandin
PKD	Polycystic kidney disease
PTH	Parathyroid hormone
RBF	Renal blood flow
RPF	Renal plasma flow
RTA	Renal tubular acidosis
SIADH	Syndrome of inappropriate ADH
SLE	Systemic lupus erythematosus
T_m	Transport maximum
UTI	Urinary tract infection

REFERENCES

1. Carlson, Bruce M. _Human Embryology and Developmental Biology : With Student Consult Access_. 3rd ed. St. Louis: Mosby, 2004.

2. Colman, Rebecca, and Ron Somogyi. _The Toronto Notes for Medical Students 2008_. New York: McGraw-Hill Medical Division, 2008.

3. Datta, Shreelata. _Renal and Urinary Systems_. Danbury: Mosby, Incorporated, 2003.

4. Field, Michael, David Harris, and Carol Pollock. _The Renal System_. New York: Churchill Livingstone, 2001.

5. Gray, Henry. _Gray's Anatomy : The Anatomical Basis of Medicine and Surgery_. Ed. Peter L. Williams. 38th ed. New York: Churchill Livingstone, 1995.

6. Guyton, Arthur C., and John E. Hall. _Textbook of Medical Physiology_. 11th ed. Philadelphia: Saunders, 2005.

7. Koeppen, Bruce M., and Bruce A. Stanton. _Renal Physiology_. 4th ed. St. Louis: Mosby, 2006.

8. Kumar, Parveen J., and Michael L. Clark, eds. _Clinical Medicine : A Textbook for Medical Students and Doctors_. Philadelphia: Saunders, 2002.

9. Kumar, Vinay, Abul K. Abbas, and Nelson Fausto. _Robbins and Cotran Pathological Basis of Disease : With Student Consult Access_. 7th ed. Philadelphia: Saunders, 2004.

10. Martin, Elizabeth A. _Concise Medical Dictionary_. New York: Oxford UP, 2003.

11. Moore, Keith L., and T. V. Persaud. _Before We Are Born : Essentials of Embryology and Birth Defects_. 6th ed. Boston: W. B. Saunders Company, 2002.

12. Moore, Keith L., Anne M. Aqur, and Arthur F. Dalley. _Essential Clinical Anatomy_. 3rd ed. Philadelphia: Lippincott Williams & Wilkins, 2006.

13. O'Callaghan, C. A. _The Renal System at a Glance_. 2nd ed. Grand Rapids: Blackwell Limited, 2006.

14. Pawlina, Wojciech, and Michael R. Ross. _Histology : A Text and Atlas with Correlated Cell and Molecular Biology_. 5th ed. Philadelphia: Lippincott Williams & Wilkins, 2006.

15. Pooler, John, and Douglas C. Eaton. _Vander's Renal Physiology_. 6th ed. New York: McGraw-Hill Scientific, Technical & Medical, 2004.

16. Sherwood, Lauralee. _Human Physiology : From Cells to Systems_. 6th ed. Belmont: Brooks/Cole, 2006.

17. Snell, Richard S. _Clinical Anatomy_. 3rd ed. Philadelphia: Lippincott Williams and Wilkins, 2007.

18. Stevens, Alan, and James S. Lowe. _Pathology : Illustrated Review in Colour_. 2nd ed. Danbury: Mosby, Incorporated, 2000.

19. Stevens, Alan, James Lowe, and Ian Scott. _Core Pathology_. 3rd ed. Edinburgh: Mosby, 2008.

20. Thomas, Robert, and Bethany Stanley. _Renal and Urinary Systems : With Student Consult Online Access_. 3rd ed. St. Louis: Mosby, 2007.

21. Voet, Donald, Judith G. Voet, and Charlotte W. Pratt. _Fundamentals of Biochemistry : Life at the Molecular Level_. New York: Wiley, 2001

Acidosis
Acid-base disturbance characterised by blood pH < 7.35 (acidaemia).

Allosteric interactions
Ligand binding at one site affects the binding of another ligand at another site (Greek: *allos,* other + *stereo,* solid or space).

Alkalosis
Acid-base disturbance characterised by blood pH > 7.45 (alkalaemia).

Anastomosis
A direct communication (natural or artificial connection) between two structures.

Arrhythmia
Any heart rhythm different from the normal (sinus rhythm).

Autoantibody
An antibody formed erroneously against one of the body's own components, as seen in autoimmune pathologies.

Calculus (pl. calculi)
A stone formed in the body, commonly in the gallbladder or urinary tract, causing pain and obstructing normal urinary flow.

Catecholamine
Group of substances functioning primarily as neurotransmitters (including adrenaline, noradrenaline and dopamine).

Creatinine
Product of creatine and creatine phosphate metabolism in muscle. Measurements of creatinine are helpful in identifying renal function, as it is normally excreted in the urine.

Cyst
Abnormal closed cavity with an epithelial lining and liquid/semi-solid contents.

Cystine
An amino acid dimer derived from the breakdown of proteins in the body. It consists of a pair of cysteine (an amino acid) molecules joined by a disulphide bond.

Cystinosis
A hereditary defect in the metabolism of amino acids, characterised by abnormal accumulation of cystine in the body.

Deamination
Metabolic process contributing to the removal of toxic nitrogenous products from the body. Deamination occurs in the liver, where the amino group $-NH_2$ is removed from an amino acid and converted to ammonia, which is metabolised to urea and excreted from the body.

Dysuria
Pain prior to, during or after passing urine.

Erythropoietin
A hormone secreted by renal mesangial and tubular cells in hypoxic states ($\downarrow O_2$ delivery to tissues). Erythropoietin stimulates red cell production in the bone marrow.

Glutaminase
An enzyme in the kidney that catalyses the breakdown of the amino acid glutamine to glutamic acid and ammonia, ultimately contributing to the production of urea.

Glycolysis
Biochemical process of glucose breakdown into lactic acid. The series of ten enzyme-catalysed reactions occurs in the cell's cytoplasm and yields energy (in the form of ATP) used for metabolic work.

Haematocrit
See PACKED CELL VOLUME.

Haematuria
Passage of blood in the urine which may be visible (macroscopic/frank haematuria), detected microscopically, or by urinalysis dipstick.

Hypoplasia
Inadequate development of an organ or tissue that is consequently smaller than average.

Intravenous
Into or within a vein (vascular compartment of the extracellular fluid).

Leukocyturia
Presence of leukocytes (white blood cells) in the urine.

Lymphoma
A malignant tumour involving lymphocytes, typically originating in lymph nodes.

Mesangium
Inner layer of the glomerulus between the glomerular capillaries.

Microalbuminuria
Excretion of a significant level of albumin in the urine (30–300 mg/24hr), not detectable with urine dipstick test strips.

Microangiopathy
Damage to small blood vessels typically leading to renal failure, haemolysis or purpura. Causative diseases include connective tissue diseases, diabetes mellitus and infections.

Packed cell volume
Fraction of the volume of whole blood occupied by red blood cells. Also known as 'haematocrit'.

Pallor
Describes the appearance of abnormally pale skin. Causes include anaemia or vasoconstriction of dermal vessels.

Pericarditis
Inflammation of the membranous sac (called the 'pericardium') which surrounds the heart.

Pitting oedema
An excess accumulation of interstitial fluid causing swelling, such that a transient indentation is left on the patient's skin after pressure with one's finger.

Plasma
The acellular component of blood, and part of the extracellular fluid compartment.

Polycythaemia
An increase in red cell volume in the blood as detected by a raised haematocrit, either because of reduction in total plasma volume (*relative* polycythaemia) or expansion of total erythrocyte volume (*absolute* polycythaemia).

Polyuria
Increased volume of dilute urine, irrespective of frequency of micturition.

Post-prandial
After eating a meal.

Proteinuria
Presence of protein in the urine.

Pyelonephritis
Infection of kidney tissue by bacterial organisms.

Renal osteodystrophy
A general term for bone disease as a result of chronic renal failure. It includes disorders such as osteoporosis, osteomalacia and osteosclerosis.

Renal threshold
The plasma concentration of a substance at which its transport maximum is reached, and the substance first starts to appear in the urine.

Septicaemia
Systemic tissue damage due to bacterial or related toxin invasion from the blood.

Shear stress
Physical force applied to the endothelium, e.g. exerted by a rise in blood pressure (this is different to the 'sheer stress' many students experience prior to exams!).

Solvent drag
Osmotically induced reabsorption of water (e.g. following Na^+ reabsorption in the proximal tubule) which leads to simultaneous transport of solutes from the ultrafiltrate into the renal interstitium. This process typically occurs in the paracellular route.

Tachycardia
In adults, a heart rate above 100 beats/min.

Tachypnoea
Increased respiratory rate. In adults, usually considered to be above 20 breaths/min.

Transport maximum
The maximum reabsorption rate for a particular substance, when all its specific carriers become saturated (fully occupied).

Uraemia
Accumulation of nitrogenous waste products such as urea in the blood (associated with uraemic acidosis).

Varicocele
Occurs when the veins of the pampiniform plexus become dilated (varicose) and tortuous, presenting as a palpable mass.

Vesico-ureteric reflux
The abnormal backflow of urine from the bladder up the ureters due to defective valves. This may lead to pyelonephritis and kidney scarring.

INDEX

A

B